WHITE BEARS

AND

OTHER UNWANTED
THOUGHTS

D1113711

DANIEL M. WEGNER

WHITE BEARS
AND
OTHER UNWANTED
THOUGHTS

*Suppression, Obsession, and the Psychology
of Mental Control*

THE GUILFORD PRESS
New York   London

Published in 1994 by The Guilford Press
A division of Guilford Publications, Inc.
72 Spring Street, New York, NY 10012

Printed in the United States of America

This book is printed on acid-free paper.

Last digit is print number: 9 8 7 6 5 4 3

Library of Congress Cataloging-in-Publication Data

Wegner, Daniel M., 1948–
    White bears and other unwanted thoughts : suppression, ob-
session, and the psychology of mental control / Daniel M. Wegner.
        p. cm.
    Reprint. Originally published: New York: Viking, 1989.
    Includes bibliographical references.
    ISBN 0-89862-223-9
    1. Thought and thinking. 2. Self-control. I. Title.
BF441.W44 1994
153.4′2—dc20   89-29505
                                                          CIP

A portion of this book first appeared in *Psychology Today.*

Grateful acknowledgment is made for permission to reprint the following material:
    Excerpts from *Human Nature and Conduct* by John Dewey.
Copyright 1922 by Henry Holt and Company and renewed 1950 by
John Dewey. Reprinted by permission of the publisher.
    Excerpt from *Letters from the Earth* by Mark Twain. Copyright
1938, 1944, 1946, ©1959, 1962 by The Mark Twain Co. Reprinted by permission of Harper & Row, Publishers, Inc.
    Excerpt from *The Analysis of Mind* by Bertrand Russell. By per-
mission of Unwin Hyman Limited.
    Excerpt from "Resolutions" from *The Complete Stories of Franz
Kafka.* Copyright ©1971 by Schocken Books, Inc. Reprinted with
permission of Schocken Books, published by Pantheon books, a division of Random House, Inc.
    Paul Zuvella quote reprinted from *Sports Illustrated,* issue of July
21, 1986. Copyright 1986 Time Inc.

For Toni

PREFACE (1994)

At the beginning, an unwanted thought is just an annoyance. You put it out of mind and it pops back suddenly later on. Despite this interruption, you try to forge ahead, to return to what you were trying to think or talk about. But then, maybe right away or maybe later, the thought intrudes once more. If you are fortunate and do the right things to dispel it, you may find that the thought eventually does stop bothering you. It goes away and the episode is over. If you make a few simple mistakes, though, ones that anyone can make under the right conditions, the thought keeps coming back again and again.

Where does it get its energy? Why does an unwanted thought sometimes return in this way—first as an annoyance, eventually as a burden, and in its extreme form to some people at some times, as a devastating affliction worse than any disease? How can a person succeed in avoiding an unwanted thought? This book presents answers to these questions that have been developed on the basis of laboratory research on thought suppression. The research suggests that the desire to suppress the thought is itself the cause of the obsession. Yes, I know this sounds wrong. It seems paradoxical indeed to blame our attempt to solve a problem for somehow creating that problem. But it turns out there is a great deal of evidence in favor of this odd power of suppression, and this book reports this evidence.

This new Guilford edition of the book is unchanged from the first edition, with the exception of this prefatory update. In these few pages, I would like to report that many things have happened since the first edition. For one, I have become a collector of objects and information related to the book. Of course, many stuffed toy white bears have made their way into my home and are now cared for by my children. People have also sent me, or I have found, enough relevant new information to fill about a foot of file drawer. Just about every major cartoon strip, for example, seems to have featured the futility of thought suppression at least once (*Calvin and Hobbes* more than that), and I have received many of these. I have also learned from several scholars all about what was an apparent Russian obsession with not thinking of white bears. Dostoevski mentioned this at one point, and of course there is the story about Tolstoy being asked as a child not to think of a white bear as well. This must have been a widespread cultural idiom in the Russia of these authors' time.

A number of other fascinating literary treatments of thought suppression have also come to my desk. People reminded me of familiar short stories by Edgar Allen Poe that illustrate the macabre obsessions that can spring from the desire to suppress a thought (*The Telltale Heart, Imp of the Perverse*). There is also a delightful story by Jorge Luis Borges called *The Zahir,* about an Argentinean coin with the noteworthy property that it cannot be put out of mind. Quotes both long and short from Mark Twain, John Steinbeck, Ernest Hemingway, and many others have arrived in the mail. And the literary repercussions of thought suppression are by no means complete. Shortly after the first edition of this book, Linda Bierds published "White Bears: Tolstoy at Astapovo" in the *New Yorker,* echoing in poetry the curious stream of consciousness of someone trying not to think.

All this literary attention has not done much to warn people away from thought suppression. The advice "just don't think about it" surfaces repeatedly anyway. In my file, for instance, is a *Time* magazine (May 1, 1989) clipping of a story that sums things up by saying: "In short, the most sensible thing to do about earth-grazing asteroids is try not to think about them." Meanwhile, several different popular psychology books (that shall remain nameless here) — including ones by some of psychology's most respected scientists — continue to recommend that people try "thought stopping" as a form of therapy for obsessions, fears, or depression. My purpose in writing this book was to tell about research that specifically calls into question the human ability to stop a thought. Even though there are some people who think this is obvious, there are others who remain unconvinced.

The research that has been conducted on thought suppression since the first edition, both in my laboratory and in a number of others around the world, has not contradicted the basic themes of this volume. We now know more details about how thought suppression operates, and we also have evidence that the same kind of ironic effects that arise from thought suppression can come from a number of other kinds of attempts to control one's mind. Attempts to concentrate, to be happy, to relax, to be good or fair, or even just to hold still, create ironic mental processes that can make us do just the opposite of these things — particularly when we are under stress or have a lot on our minds. Just as the white bear comes back, so do many of the other thoughts and mental states we hope to push away — apparently, just because we are in fact trying to avoid them. The scientific evidence continues to accumulate, in other words, to verify the ideas presented in these pages.

I have formed the distinct impression that the book serves several audiences, as I have now heard from members of each. I wrote it originally for the general reader, whoever this lucky person may be, thinking that everyone has unwanted thoughts and that observations on this might be both interesting and helpful. The plan also was to make the book useful to my colleagues in psychology, as a reference and as an initial guide to research and theory in this area. I was hoping to get the topic of thought suppression into the headlights of other scientific psychologists who might be intrigued by the research problems and take over the study of them where my work has fallen short. I am not sure in retrospect that I planned, however, to try to make the book as useful as it seems to be. Enough psychological practitioners—clinical psychologists, psychiatrists, and other psychotherapists—have called and written to report using the book as a basis for their psychotherapeutic suggestions that I am now convinced it can be of service in this way.

The audience I am most pleased to serve with this book is the group of people who have significant problems with unwanted thoughts. Calls and letters have come to me from many quarters reporting relief from symptoms, insights into problems, and other heartening responses to the book, and I am delighted at these. (I view these endorsements with some skepticism, however, as I fully realize that very few readers who found the book useless or dreary would take the trouble to get in touch with me to report this.) The stories I have heard tend to be testimonials that suggest there is something very useful here to people suffering from fears or phobias, thoughts that are sad or depressing, strange thoughts, thoughts of immoral or undesirable acts, thoughts of suicide, thoughts of unwanted movements (even a problem in a golf swing, for example), or garden-variety thoughts of fattening foods, alcohol, or other addictions.

Let me remind you, though, that this is not a self-help book. I do not offer any 5-point plans or other specific recommendations. My approach as a scientist is simply to investigate the nature and consequences of thought suppression. Sometimes, however, learning that suppression causes obsession can be quite enlightening about one's own obsessions, and this may be the main way in which this book is self-helpful. With this in mind, let me then put aside my file folders and invite you to continue reading. Please join me on a scientific journey through one of the mind's most fundamental peculiarities—its profound inability to stop itself.

D. M. W.
Charlottesville, Virginia
February, 1994

PREFACE

You would think this book was about white bears, given the title and all. And in a way, it is. Although the topic is really unwanted thoughts and how people try to control them, white bears come into the picture because of a story about the young Tolstoy. It seems he was once challenged by his older brother to stand in a corner until he could stop thinking of a white bear. Of course, he stood there confused for some time. And the point was made: We do not seem to have much control over our minds, especially when it comes to suppressing thoughts that are unwanted.

I ran across that story some years ago, and it must have impressed me. After all, I have written an entire book about it. The topic, moreover, is something of a departure from my more typical research and writing in psychology. As a social psychologist, my general focus is the study of social cognition—how people think about themselves and others. So, for example, I have been concerned with how self-awareness works, how individuals understand their actions, and how social relationships influence thinking and memory. Off and on in the study of these things, though, I have puzzled at the human inability to say no. When we admonish ourselves not to do something, not to believe something, not to feel something, even not to think something, our attempt to say no is often no more effective than a flyswatter held up to stop a cannonball.

My interest in this odd human problem was piqued, perhaps permanently, by the results of a little experiment conducted in my laboratory. Borrowing directly from Tolstoy's curious exploit, the experiment called for people to report everything that came to mind as they tried not to think of a white bear. And just like the child stymied in the corner, most everyone reported thinking repeatedly of a white bear. There were yet other noteworthy results of the experiment that intrigued me even more—but then, I am getting ahead of myself. We have an entire book before us in which to learn about this remarkable puzzle.

Suffice it to say that the study points up a general human problem in the area of mental control. We desire, sometimes very profoundly and desperately, to be able to control our thoughts. We may wish not to think of many things: a loved one's death, an upcoming dental procedure, the thought of food when we are dieting, the idea of doing something stupid or harmful, visions of smoking or drinking alcohol or of some other habit we are hoping to control, or perhaps thoughts of a time when we were victimized, humiliated, or betrayed. Although it may seem silly to suppress the thought of a white bear, mental control is serious business. Obsessions, addictions, depression, and panic—states of mind distinguished for their inner turmoil—are what we encounter in the struggle against the thoughts that we truly desire not to have. Obviously, mental control is a key to mental peace, and we will need to study it in depth if we hope ever to understand how to do it effectively.

Oddly, the topic of mental control is not yet a standard subject for scientific psychology. There are hundreds of books about how the mind works, and even more on psychotherapeutic recommendations for overcoming distress, but mental control appears only on the fringes. The idea that we can control what we think, or at least that we often try to do so, is thus a fresh focal point for investigation. As it turns out, many of the great dead psychologists expressed fascinating opinions about mental control, many studies that have been done for other purposes are highly relevant to mental control, and some of the most recent breakthroughs in cognitive science, the psychology of emotion, cognitive therapy, and yes, even my old friend social cognition, provide sparkling insights on the topic as well. This book brings these things together, along with a number of more recent white bear studies done in my laboratory, in an attempt to make a first foothold for the psychological study of mental control.

I would like to thank my coauthors on the first white bear studies—Dave Schneider, Sam Carter, and Teri White—for bearing with me. I am also grateful to my colleagues and friends who were kind enough to read this manuscript or parts of it and make helpful suggestions. They include Chris Gilbert, Dan Gilbert, Jamie Pennebaker, Dave Schneider, Bill Swann, Abe Tesser, Sonya Trubshaw, Robin Vallacher, Toni Wegner, Rich Wenzlaff, and Robert Wicklund. Finally, I owe a debt to Trinity University for providing a semester leave during which I could work on this book full time.

D. M. W.
San Antonio, Texas

CONTENTS

ONE

Mental Control

The highest possible stage in moral culture is when we recognize that we ought to control our thoughts.

—Charles Darwin, *The Descent of Man*

When I first learned there was such a thing as an indelible pencil (I think it was in third grade) I was overwhelmed. Its purplish marks could *never be erased*. This finality was too much for my young sensibilities. Erasing was my life, the center of a daily eternity of smudges, errors, and regret played out under the eye of my teacher, a universal master of human penmanship. As it happened, of course, I learned that many things are as good as indelible, from bounced checks to auto wrecks, and I have come to accept this as a necessary part of life on earth.

There is still one slight problem. Although reality can't be erased, it seems only fair that our *thoughts* about things might be erasable. We can change our mind, get new ideas, see things in different ways, and easily move our attention from one thing to another. In other words, it usually seems that we can control what we think. When we try not to think about something, though, our thoughts can be as indelible as the marks made by that purple pencil. Unwanted thoughts—about food when we're on a diet, about that little lump that could be cancer, about a lost love whose absence we grieve, even about the mutton-headed thing we said to the boss yesterday—often seem etched permanently in our mind. The silliest little thought can be this way. Try right now, for instance, not to think of a white bear.

1

Really. Put down the book and look away and stop thinking of a white bear. I'm serious. Try it.

The White Bear. Welcome back. How successful were you? Did you avoid a white bear for a few seconds or a minute? Did it return to your mind even once after you had wished it away? Most people report one or more returns, and some of them also stop at this point and remark that it is a cute trick, maybe good for a full minute of entertainment at children's birthday parties. There may be something to learn, however, on taking seriously the observation that people do not do a good job of avoiding an unwanted thought, even a warm fuzzy one like a white bear.

An experiment was conducted in which people were asked not to think of a white bear.[1] Each person was isolated in a laboratory room, seated at a table with a microphone and with a bell like the one at a hotel desk. The person was asked to spend five minutes saying everything that came to mind into the microphone. One or two people complained that nothing came to mind, but most of them did a fine job of yammering on about this and that for the full time period. They described the walls, talked about lunch, and often got into extended monologues on their families or jobs or future plans.

At the end of this period, the experimenter came in and asked the person to continue—but this time, not to think of a white bear. If the thought of a white bear came up anyway, the person was to ring the bell and go on. On the average, people in this predicament rang the bell more than 6 times in the next five minutes and mentioned white bear out loud several times as well. Below is the transcript of the recording made by one such person, a female college student. As you can see, she had a frustrating time trying to remove the unwanted thought from her mind, rang the bell 15 times, and never really succeeded in the whole five minutes she tried.

Of course now the only thing I'm going to think about is a white bear. Okay, I mean it's hard to think that I can see a bell* . . . and don't think about a white bear. Ummm, what was I thinking of before? See, if I think about flowers a lot* . . . I'll think about a white bear, it's impossible.* I could ring this bell over and over* and over* and over* and . . . a white bear* . . . and okay . . . so, my fingernails are really bad they . . . ummm . . . they need to be painted because they are . . . ummm . . . they're chipping at the ends. One thing about this is every time that I really want like . . . ummm . . . to talk, think, to not think* about the white bear, then it makes me think about the white bear more so it doesn't work, so I'm going to try harder not to think about the white bear. Okay, it's like I have to force myself to not think* about the white bear. So, I also have this little brown freckle on my finger and I also have little sparklies* all over my hands and neck from Halloween last night 'cause we got all dressed up and went out and it was pretty fun. We were, we were . . . ummm . . . people from Venus, who were all in purple and . . . (sigh) . . . we painted our hair purple and glittery and . . . ummm . . . made it look real weird. (Pause) And I'm trying to think of a million things to make me think about everything* but a white bear and I keep thinking of it over* and over* and over* and over. So . . . ummm, hey, look at this brown wall. It's like every time I try and not think about a white bear, I'm still thinking about one, and I'm tired of ringing the bell. So, instead I'm going to think about relaxing my toes and getting all the tension out of there and then relaxing my feet and getting all the tension out of my feet. I'm trying to make the tension go away, sweeping it out through imagery. I'm upset but . . . because (pause) but all I think about is white bear.* Apparently when I have to keep talking, I think . . . I don't know.

*Indicates a bell ring. She was instructed to ring a bell each time the thought came to mind.

Eventually, of course, people do drift off to something else and stop returning to the white bear. But even then, the problem of thought suppression is not solved. Some of the people in this experiment were asked immediately after this session to continue for yet another five-minute period. But now, however, their task was to *think* of a white bear. These people became unusually preoccupied with white bear thoughts, ringing the bell 16 times and mentioning a white bear 14 times. This level of thinking is unusual because people who are simply asked to think about a white bear from the outset report thinking about it quite a bit less (12 rings and 11 mentions). The people thinking about a white bear after suppressing it tended even to show an *acceleration* of white bear thoughts over time. The irony, then, is not only that people found it hard to suppress a thought in the first place, but that the attempt to do this made them especially inclined to become absorbed with the thought later on.

Why *shouldn't* we be able to suppress a thought? Suppression seems like a simple, obvious, and important ability, as basic as thinking itself, and we don't seem to have it. Imagine—we are drawn to the very item we are attempting to avoid, clambering desperately away from the thought only to stumble back upon it again and again. Like a moth drawn to a flame, or a chicken entranced by a line drawn in the dirt, the person attempting to avoid an unwanted thought doesn't seem very smart. We can do so much—our minds so flexible and imaginative and complex—but all the IQ points in the world don't keep us from puzzling repeatedly over one thought.

This book is about this strange puzzle, the problem of influencing one's own mental activities. It turns out the puzzle is tremendously complicated, a labyrinth of exciting clues, dead ends, and odd pathways that occasionally shuttles would-be solvers off to Mars, Cleveland, and elsewhere. We hope to keep away from such places in this book, so we will follow a fairly straight path toward the solution. Still, before we're done, we will consult ideas arising from cognitive psychology, psychiatry, artificial intelligence, social psychology, psychophysiology, clinical psychology, and even philosophy and mathematics. To begin looking into these matters, we'll consider in this chapter several key ideas underlying the analysis of mental control.

Worry and Distress. The need for mental control probably would not occur to us if we had no worries or problems. If everything in life went well, we would seldom take time to reflect on our emotions or thought processes, or even our actions. We would be too busy having fun. We attempt mental control primarily when we have the feeling that something is wrong or soon will be. Mental control usually starts from an exasperated attempt to deal with something unpleasant, and the mental turmoil we usually discover when we step into the white bear trap makes things worse yet.

This happens all too often, for it seems unwanted thoughts can arise from many possible sources. If we are concerned about an upcoming event (say, our wedding), if we cannot get over something that happened a while ago (for example, our home was robbed), or if we cannot seem to make ourselves behave as we wish (stopping smoking, perhaps), we will probably have unwanted thoughts lurking about. Whether we are trying to deal with fears, phobias, obsessions, addictions, traumas, confusions, or just garden-variety worries, we find that we can't seem to change the channel on the mental TV. Unwanted thoughts can be especially lasting when they represent unwanted realities, things we cannot change. Like Jimmy Swaggart, the televangelist who admitted "moral failure" when a prostitute came forward to claim she posed nude for him, we want the reality to go away. In his words, "I wish it were possible to erase the ledger and start over again. But of course it is not."[2]

When an unwanted thought is with us, there may be little peace. The vaguely satisfied and peaceful state that occurs just as we wake up in the morning lasts a moment. Then, however, we begin to review for ourselves where we are and what we're doing—and the unwanted thought bursts into view. If it is severe enough, we may even shudder as it hits, and then watch in dread as the empty optimism of sleep drops away and the unwanted thought settles over us for another day. If the thought is something we can set aside for a while, we do so and begin our routine. But the naive freshness of that morning moment is gone, and we know there is something on our mind that will not depart.

We need not always have the *same* unwanted thought every day. It is just that on most days, we have a "most unwanted" one to report. My wife and I were going to Florida on vacation, for instance, and had planned to rent a convertible and soak up some sun. The day we were leaving, a good friend came back from a dermatology appointment sporting several small scars where minor skin cancers had been removed. He casually pointed to a spot on my arm and said, "Hey, that's just like one of them." This totally ruined my vacation. I swam only at dusk to avoid the sun, kept the convertible top up every day, and thought about skin cancer every few minutes. As our car neared Disney World and my wife gleefully pointed to the Magic Kingdom, I could only say, "Yes, dear, but that's not important now." This one unwanted thought hijacked my mind for ten days, and then departed (when I got home and saw a dermatologist—who, of course, laughed). Looking back at this, I can laugh too, but at the time I was deep in despair and not much was funny at all.

Most people report having at least one thought that won't go away. In a study conducted early in this century, one psychologist found that many of the students in his classes admitted to having "fixed ideas" that could not be eliminated.[3] In a San Antonio study, when 180 people were asked to write down an unwanted thought, almost every person had one or more to mention.[4] They reported that their thought was "distressing," and occurred from once a day to every few minutes. Similarly, researchers in England report that people have "normal" obsessions that parallel in several ways the "abnormal" obsessions individuals seek psychotherapy to eliminate.[5] The fact that most people report such thoughts may provide a bit of solace to those of us who think we're odd for worrying. But this fact also indicates that there is indeed a general human problem in the area of mental control.

Unwanted thoughts turn up in a variety of psychological disorders. Of course, they are in center stage when people suffer from obsessions (recurrent unwanted thoughts) or compulsions (recurrent unwanted actions). But having trouble with thoughts that won't go away is characteristic also in many cases of depression, phobic or anxiety reactions, posttraumatic stress disorders, self-control problems such as addictions and eating disorders, and even in psychotic reactions such as schizophrenia. It is not surprising that mental control is rare when people have very severe problems, because the extremes of mental disorder are almost defined in terms of control lapses. However, unwanted thoughts themselves do not define a particular form of psychological disorder. Rather, they occur at all points in the spectrum from normal to abnormal, cutting across different kinds of disorders rather than distinguishing them from one another. Unwanted thoughts are a general symptom of mental distress, a painful intrusion for anyone. So it is important to understand these everyday glimmerings of madness in us all.

Freud and the Dark Side. Sigmund Freud recognized the deep and abiding desire people have to erase certain of their thoughts, and he insisted that people are commonly able to do this. According to his psychoanalytic theory, we keep the darker side of our minds hidden, not only from others but from ourselves. His idea of *repression*—the erasure of thoughts from memory—is the most major recognition of the problem of mental control in the history of psychology.[6]

It is debatable whether Freud would himself have portrayed repression as a process of mental control. He described people as being *driven* to try to forget painful or unappealing thoughts, and he argued that often people manage to forget without even knowing that they have forgotten. Freud described the process of repression as largely unconscious, unavailable for inspection by the person who does it. So, for example, Freud held that many of our childhood memories—about nursing, toilet training, masturbation, and relationships with our parents—are sufficiently disturbing for us to want to forget them. Thus, we both forget them and indeed even forget the act of forgetting itself. Freud said this is why we can't remember much of our early childhood.

Naturally, getting clear evidence of such repression is difficult. You can't just ask people if they ever repressed anything, because by definition they will have forgotten both what they repressed and that they repressed it. Determining whether repression really happens, then, is much like finding out whether the refrigerator light stays on when you close the door. Perhaps for this reason, the concept of repression has not held up too well in the large number of scientific investigations that have been aimed at it since Freud's day. Although studies show that our memory systems are complex and may sometimes hide things from us, the research does not offer support for a strong version of Freud's claim—that we *usually* forget painful or distressing ideas.[7] If anything, it shows instead that our memories are remarkably resistant to deletion.

Memory, however, may not be the issue. Although Freud focused on it, and led many investigators along the same path, it is probably not the key arena for the activity of mental control. Suppose, for instance, that you have some unwanted thought—say, an upcoming dental appointment. For Freud's classical version of repression to occur, you would have to forget this appointment. In fact, you would have to forget it so completely that you would be surprised and deny all knowledge of it if someone tried to remind you. This probably happens once in a while, but not too often or most dentists would be out of business. Instead of forgetting the dentist, you will just not think about the dentist. You will put it out of mind—not by erasing it permanently from memory, but rather by keeping it temporarily from your conscious thoughts.

This is the difference between Freud's early theories of mental control and the topic of this book. We are not particularly interested in repression (the erasure of memory), but rather in suppression (avoiding consciousness of a thought). Repression implies that we could never get the thought back, whereas suppression suggests only that we're not thinking of it. After all, we avoid consciousness of thoughts all the time, whereas real memory loss seems to occur only under extreme conditions (when people have amnesia resulting from physical or psychological trauma, or have their memories changed while they are under hypnosis).[8] To be fair, we should point out that Freud described conscious suppression and related processes as well. Going back to being unfair, we can note that his emphasis on the repression of memory may have led to one of the bigger wild goose chases in the history of psychology. There has been an unresolved controversy for years about whether repression ever occurs, how much it happens, and how it should be tested, and not much in the way of solid evidence has come of any of it.

Still, it is clear that Freud started one idea that continues to gather momentum: Mental control can backfire. The things people try not to think about can come back to haunt them. Freud held that repressions in early childhood, and even later, can form the seed for subsequent anxiousness, guilt, distress, and even physical and psychological symptoms of many kinds.[9] This idea is echoed in a wide range of more modern findings. People who try not to think about their grief over a lost loved one, for example, can take the longest time to get over their loss.[10] Surgery patients who try not to think about their upcoming operation can become the most upset about it afterwards.[11] Incest victims who try to block out the thoughts of their victimization can become particularly obsessed and tormented by their memories of what happened.[12] People who try not to think of food while on a diet can later become so preoccupied with food that they go on eating binges and become overweight.[13] Those of us who hide our secrets and suppress our thoughts about traumatic events in our past can become ill—not just with psychological illnesses, but with physical disease as well.[14]

It is not always the case, however, that suppression leads to such unfortunate consequences. Sometimes it is the only thing one can do, and sometimes it has no appreciable impact on our future lives. But, like the white bear thoughts that come back at a high rate once suppression is over, our thoughts about anything that was once suppressed may return to overtake our minds and preoccupy our thinking. Although Freud's recognition of this possibility is only a part of the modern outlook on mental control, he must be credited for alerting us to the dangers that lurk in the shadows when we attempt to put our minds in the dark.

James and the Lighter Side. The power of the will was something that deeply impressed William James, the founder of American psychology. He thought people could do marvelous things, if only they had the willpower. The phenomenon of will was worthy of study, as he saw it, because eventually its influence over human action might be predicted and understood. Instead of taking the Freudian view that mental control is something we do to struggle with our internal devils, however, he perceived a nobler purpose to it all, a version of mental control shaped from optimism and a "can-do" approach.

James held that the basic feature of will is "effort of attention."[15] By this he meant that we do things on purpose by directing our attention to some idea of what we will do. We open a can of tuna by attending to the thought of opening the can, for instance, and what makes this "willful" is the fact that it takes effort to direct our attention. Mental control thus precedes all other kinds of voluntary control—control over our actions, our emotions, our thoughts themselves. To the degree that we can do anything at all on purpose, we do it by willfully moving our attention toward what it is we wish to do.

James admitted freely, of course, that there are plenty of

psychological events over which people have no control at all. So, although we may sometimes effortfully direct our attention, it can as well be pushed around by forces we cannot control. This idea has been echoed in modern psychology by a distinction between automatic and controlled processes of thought.[16] Automatic processes take little conscious attention, as when we "automatically" read simple road signs and billboards as we pass them or attend to a loud noise; we don't have to concentrate on what we are doing. Controlled processes take a lot of attention, as when we try to read a difficult textbook or listen in on a quiet conversation; we have to concentrate all our attention on the task to get it done. Both automatic and controlled activities can certainly be classed as varieties of "thinking," but the first is effortless while the second takes willful work. Mental control, in the sense we will use it in this book, is happening only in the second case, when we are consciously controlling our attention.

James is also known for naming the "stream of consciousness." He remarked on the seamless, flowing quality of our mental lives, noting that we always have something on our minds. Part of James's upbeat approach was to emphasize that the control of this flow occurs in the movement of attention toward things (rather than away). So, in contrast to Freud's focus on the "unwantedness" of some thoughts, James was more concerned with *wanted* thoughts. He saw the control of the stream of consciousness as a positive enterprise, a sighting toward friendly ports that at worst might only be hard to find. This view of mental control indicates that *concentration* could be the only important problem we face. He emphasized that to concentrate on one idea, all we need to do is keep competing ideas from coming to mind.

With this realization, we can now see that concentration and suppression are opposite sides of the same coin. Whenever we exercise our wills, it is by *moving* our attention. Such movement means we are both moving toward something and moving away from something else. Concentration is the moving toward, and suppression is the moving away. So, suppression implies concentration; in suppressing the thought of an upcoming visit from our mother-in-law, for instance, we distract ourselves by concentrating on something else more pleasant—say, the nuclear waste problem. The use of concentration as a means of suppression is exactly what the participant in the white bear study was trying to do; she was attempting to think of other things as her way of getting away from the white bear.

To concentrate, in turn, we have to suppress competing thoughts. When we wish to think about something clearly and well, we must set aside potential distractions and not think of them. It is interesting that when we use these processes of concentration and suppression to control our minds, we seem to focus on only one at a time, purposefully controlling one and letting the other follow. We might purposefully concentrate on the intricacies of an income tax form, for example, and to do this it happens we must suppress thoughts of going out for pizza. Or we might purposefully suppress the unwanted thought of an upcoming awkward confrontation with someone, and in order to do this concentrate on a television show. Concentration and suppression are just two different views of the same underlying process of mental control—the willful movement of attention.

This book concentrates more on suppression than on concentration. Clearly, we must understand both to get a firm grip on mental control. We cannot concentrate well without suppressing, and we cannot suppress well without concentrating. But lapses of concentration are seldom as disturbing and intrusive as lapses of suppression. Unwanted thoughts can fill us with horror and rule our lives, whereas problems in concentration only leave us unfocused and confused. It seems important to examine suppression more closely than concentration, perhaps because the darker side of anything is more mysterious than the lighter side.

Dewey and the Practical Side. The philosopher and educator

John Dewey was convinced, with Freud and James, that we can control our minds.[17] He added a key idea to their analyses, however, a practical and down-to-earth idea that makes Freud and James look like the brothers Grimm, spinners of fairy tales. Dewey explained that we can't just wish our minds to go in one direction or another, to concentrate or to suppress, without the necessary practice, know-how, and skill. Freud thought we could suppress, and James thought we could concentrate, but neither of them fully realized how hard it is to do these things, and how tricky and unexpected the results can be.

Think of what happens when you are lolling in bed on a holiday morning and you resolve to get up. Ten minutes later, you resolve again. "Okay, I'm getting up *now*," you say to yourself, and you sink slightly deeper in the bed. This can go on forever, it seems, and you wonder whether your attempts at control are even real—or just illusions, sugarplums that dance through your head without getting anything sticky. A similar sequence occurs when you are trying to lose weight, and you head for the food late at night. All the while you are saying to yourself, "Don't do this. This will keep you fat. Hold everything. Stop. I mean it." You then eat large amounts of whatever is available. All the willpower you can muster is insufficient to keep you from your old haunts and habits.

Exactly the same thing can occur when you are trying to control your thoughts. You want to concentrate on a speaker, for instance, and instead you keep drifting to think of the sunshine streaming through the window or the air conditioning blowing on your neck. You want to suppress the thought of a plane crash as you board a flight, and instead you keep thinking of what a crash would be like, or what your family would do without you. Your attempts at mental control can be totally worthless, a little voice in your head wailing against the forward marching of the rest of your mind. It is not as easy as Freud and James imagined it to be, and Dewey recognized this as the center of the problem.

He made this point very nicely in *Human Nature and Conduct:*

> Recently a friend remarked to me that there was one superstition current among even cultivated persons. They suppose that if one is told what to do, if the right *end* is pointed to them, all that is required in order to bring about the right act is will or wish on the part of the one who is to act. He used as an illustration the matter of physical posture; the assumption that if a man is told to stand up straight, all that is further needed is wish and effort on his part, and the deed is done. He pointed out that this belief is on a par with primitive magic in its neglect of attention to the means which are involved in reaching an end. And he went on to say that the prevalence of this belief, starting with false notions about the control of the body and extending to control of mind and character, is the greatest bar to intelligent social progress. (p. 28)

> Of course something happens when a man acts upon his idea of standing straight. For a little while, he stands differently, but only a different kind of badly. He then takes the unaccustomed feeling which accompanies his unusual stand as evidence that he is now standing right. But there are many ways of standing badly, and he has simply shifted his usual way to a compensatory bad way at some opposite extreme. When we realize this fact, we are likely to suppose that it exists because control of the *body* is physical and hence is external to mind and will. Transfer the command inside character and mind, and it is fancied that an idea of an end and the desire to realize it will take immediate effect. After we get to the point of recognizing that habits must intervene between wish and execution in the case of bodily acts, we still cherish the illusion that they can be dispensed with in the case of mental and moral acts. (p. 29)

We clearly need effective means, what Dewey would call habits, if we hope to control our minds. We cannot hope to influence our unwanted thoughts or even our wanted ones if we don't know how, and all our efforts will be fruitless. We usually seem to fool ourselves in this regard, thinking that we can simply "be different" and therefore change. So, we make New Year's resolutions, for instance, to stop smoking, lose weight, get along better with others, stop drinking so much, control our tempers, and so on. The resolve may have some influence at first, but more often than not, if we happen to remember a few months later that we even resolved something, we realize quickly that the resolution fell through.

In one study of New Year's resolutions, 60 percent of them were broken in six months.[18] This study polled people who called in after a television appeal for participants in research on resolutions. The participants were sufficiently motivated to go to this trouble, and so may have been more successful than the rest of us, who resolve quietly, to ourselves, to "be better." Research of this kind therefore probably even overestimates the degree to which our wishes about ourselves come true. Wishing alone is not usually enough. To control what we are, what we think, and how we feel, takes work. We need to learn what to do, not just want to do it.

The illusion that people can change at will is very seductive. This is particularly true when it is *other* people who need to change. It is easy to stand in judgment of someone who is being wrong or stupid, and insist that just a little willpower would fix everything. This is the standpoint that Nancy Reagan voiced in her "Just say no" program, a uniquely unsophisticated campaign against drug abuse. This program assumed that if people haven't tried something, the pressure on them to do it is imaginary, and they can just decide not to. If it were really that easy, however, everyone would have already said no and left Nancy reminding them to say "Thank you," too. When we look at others behaving in ways we wish they would control, it can appear that their only problem is lack of backbone. It is only when we focus this kind of demand on ourselves that we begin to learn how hard it can be to change a person through will alone. Habitual thoughts and emotions may very well not listen as we "just say no," and it may be necessary to turn to a variety of more subtle techniques.

A Preview of the Book. In collecting the basic ideas of James, Freud, and Dewey to introduce this book, it is clear we are taking a very Western approach to the mind. The notion that the mind can and should be controlled is part of our cultural and historical tradition, and although there are counterparts in Eastern thought, they are different in many ways. Most notably, mental control is typically treated as a religious and mystical phenomenon in these philosophies rather than as a personal problem or concern of psychological science.[19] In the West, however, we use science on everything—with considerable success—and it seems natural to extend this approach to the question of the self-control of thought and emotion.

The research and ideas presented in these pages explore how people deal with unwanted thoughts, and what the pitfalls can be when their efforts take particular forms. In this sense, it is meant to be a field manual for dealing with unwanted thoughts in the wild. Although there will be no step-by-step lessons and no quick solutions, there will be information on what can go right and what can go wrong when we try to control our minds. With any luck, we may draw some ideas from this to help us understand and control ourselves more appropriately and effectively. At least, we may become better able to recognize situations in which attempts at mental control are likely to be themselves a problem.

The following chapters explore the use of mental control in the struggle against unwanted thoughts. A key question to begin with is why people suppress thoughts at all. Learning something about *why* and *when* we exercise mental control is one way to gain a sense of what it is, so we will examine the wellsprings of suppression in Chapter 2. The more critical question for many of us who are antsy to hurry up and suppress a thought, of course, is *how* suppression proceeds, and this is the focus of the next large segment of the book. Chapter 3 examines the mental mechanics underlying the act of thought suppression. It looks at how the mind is constructed, and at how the special format of this mental apparatus may constrain our abilities to suppress.

A concern with how we suppress is also present in Chapter 4, but in this case the emphasis is less mechanical and more on what it looks like from inside the head of someone who is suppressing. What people really do to suppress a thought is to think of something else, and this chapter is about the operation of this process of self-distraction. In Chapter 5, we examine how people engage in external processes of self-distraction—by changing their surroundings. Not all mental control goes on inside the head, and there are many ways we can guide ourselves to concentrate or suppress merely by making changes in where we are and what we're looking at.

The next section of the book examines psychological processes that are influenced by thought suppression. So, in passing from questions of why and when and how, we come to focus on the question of *with what effect* suppression occurs. Chapter 6 inquires whether it is possible to change our beliefs and attitudes by the willful control of thinking, and as we shall see, there are often cases in which such change is hard to manage. Chapter 7 addresses another potential consequence of thought suppression—our ability to change our moods by changing our minds. Here the concern is with using mental control to avoid unwanted emotions such as sadness. The related problem we explore in Chapter 8 is how mental control impinges on unwanted emotions such as anxiety and agitation. We will take a careful look at how suppression can influence our bodily symptoms and emotional experience.

The last chapter of the book takes up a theme that resurfaces at many points—the idea that suppression can create obsessions. Our concern in these final pages is with discerning when suppression is the solution to a problem, and when it is itself the problem. It is possible to suppress too little, and to suppress too much. In this book, we will try to discover how to suppress when we need to, and just how much suppression it is good to have.

TWO

Wellsprings of Suppression

We have a power to suspend the prosecution of this or that desire; as everyone may daily experiment in himself. This seems to me the source of all liberty.

—John Locke, *An Essay Concerning Human Understanding*

Some things are just plain disgusting. There's no need to make a list of them here, because that itself would be disgusting. But you know what I'm talking about. Insects, for example. Vomit, too. This is starting to sound like that list already, so I'd better quit. The point is there are some things that are universally repugnant, and we all know what they are. People in one study, for instance, were asked to pour some orange juice from a carton, put the carton back in the refrigerator, and then watch as a (dried) cockroach was placed in the glass of juice.[20] Of course they wouldn't drink that juice. But many of them wouldn't even drink from a different, new glass of juice poured later from the same carton that had been used to fill the tainted glass. The cockroach is so disgusting that it "rubs off" on things it didn't even touch.

Then again, think of children. They sometimes eat mud, carry frogs in their pockets, and even write on the walls with the contents of their diapers. They don't seem to understand what is disgusting until they find out from us, the wise (and disgusted) adults. Unwanted thoughts work just like disgusting things.

Although it often seems that we know exactly which thoughts nobody should want, it turns out someone wants them. Some people *like* to dwell on death and blood. Some people *like* to reminisce about that time their lover was unfaithful. Some people *like* cockroaches and keep them in collections, pinned like butterflies, so they can think about them all the time. The thoughts we personally find detestable can even change from day to day, and we begin to wonder just what it is that makes some thoughts unwanted and others welcome.

This chapter is about this question. The concern is with the wellsprings of suppression, what it is that leads us to try not to think of things. We will begin by considering the kinds of thoughts people report they don't want to have. Our more central preoccupation, though, will be with the particular settings people get into that can make almost any thought unwanted. The question of interest here is what kinds of situations or predicaments might lead anyone (including you or me) not to want a particular thought. Although we can't change who we are, we can sometimes choose the situations we enter. In so choosing, we may have some liberty to influence the very beginning of the mental control process—the things we wish to suppress in the first place. If we can avoid the situations that prompt us to suppress, we can bypass the difficulties that suppression can produce.

The Most Unwanted List. What thoughts do people express the desire to avoid? The contents of such a list will vary, of course, with the time and customs of the people, with their sex and age and habitat. In 1903 in France, for example, the renowned psychiatrist Pierre Janet reported the obsessions of his patients in five major groups: sacrilegious thoughts, urges to commit crimes, shame about one's behavior, shame about one's body, and hypochondria.[21] These obsessions are thoughts that the people believed they were thinking *too much,* and so qualify as very unwanted. Many of these topics are still favorites today, and clinical psychologists now listing the obsessions of their patients typically include categories such as self-doubt, fear of social inadequacy, moral shame, shame about one's physique, health worries, concerns about bodily functions, worry about death, fear of dirt and contamination, concern about possible harm to self or others, sexual thoughts, aggressive thoughts, and concern with orderliness and cleanliness.[22]

These lists come only from studies of people who have such severe problems with unwanted thoughts that they seek psychotherapy. What about everyone else? Far fewer studies of unwanted thoughts have been conducted among those who are not severely afflicted by them, but this research indicates a similar pattern. Several studies of the unwanted thoughts reported by college students in Texas, for example, revealed the following major categories, in order from more to less frequent: problems in relationships (jealousy, being jilted, arguing, loneliness), school worries (failing, not getting things done), general worries about life and the future, death of loved ones, fear of being victimized (rape, robbery), lack of money, physical appearance, sexual impulses, health, food and eating, and repeating songs.[23]

Among adults studied in England, several similar themes arise.[24] The people in this study were encouraged to reveal any intrusive, unacceptable thoughts or impulses they had, and the things they volunteered thus tended to include more unwanted *actions* than the other lists. Their unwanted action impulses included such things as becoming violent during sex, jumping on the tracks as a train approaches, shouting at someone, crashing the car on purpose, saying rude things to people, sexually assaulting someone, and jumping from the top of a tall building. The unwanted thoughts included such things as an accident occurring to a loved one, food calorie content, a humiliating experience many years ago, and wishing someone dead.

After seeing these collections of unwanted thoughts, you can rest assured that your own probably fit in perfectly well.

Everyone appears to think strange things, sometimes *very* strange things, and wish the thoughts would go away. The question is, Why these thoughts and not others? One general theory is just that unwanted thoughts are unpleasant, leading to negative emotions such as fear, guilt, shame, anxiety, sadness, or disgust. This was the way Freud envisioned thought suppression and repression. He believed that people do not want to have thoughts that make them feel bad, and so he transformed the problem of unwanted thoughts into the problem of unwanted feelings.

Freud's theory of emotions is very deep and complex, and probably right in just about as many ways as it is wrong. He believed that certain thoughts were attached to unpleasant feelings because the thoughts were reminiscent of battles we have as children between our desires and our realities. Reality—in the form of parents and society—prevents us from doing many of the things that feel good, from constant suckling to free-form bowel evacuation and public masturbation. The battles that make us inhibit these things can leave wounds that do not heal, particularly if they were hard-fought or too easily won. Hence, later in life we may find that thoughts even distantly related to certain of these themes can make us uneasy. A child who experienced a harsh toilet training, for instance, may be excessively worried about messiness as an adult. Many of our unwanted thoughts as adults may seem totally divorced from childhood themes, but Freud would insist that there is always some connection.

This theory makes some sense if you read it carefully and think about it for a while.[25] There is some modern evidence for certain aspects of the theory, and research continues to reveal observations consistent with or at least broadly suggested by the theory.[26] It is too cumbersome and multifaceted, however, for most everyday unwanted thoughts. If someone has unwanted thoughts about a spouse dying, for example, Freudian theory could probably interpret that in many ways—a different way, perhaps, for each person who has such a thought. For one, the thoughts might represent a wish for the spouse to die. For another, they might come from a wish for the spouse to survive. And in either case, it would probably be argued that the real motive is not aimed at the spouse at all but arises instead because the spouse is being treated as a mental stand-in for Mom or Dad or someone else.

The difficulty, then, is in knowing which of the explanations—all of which arise from the same theory—is the one for which the theory should be held accountable. Squabbles among psychoanalysts on such points usually take the form of readings from Freud and discussions of what he "really meant" in the thousands of different ideas in his voluminous writings. In the end, the theory turns out to be a marvelous interpretive device, a way of giving meaning to past events. But its very richness makes it a poor predictive device, and thus it lends little meaning to future events. It doesn't usually make clear what will happen next. A predictive theory of unwanted thoughts can be developed only if we wish in the meantime to run roughshod over much of Freud's approach. We can only agree with him on a basic idea—that there is an emotional reaction often attached to the occurrence of unwanted thoughts.

Grinding to a Halt.   The crux of the matter is not emotion, but rather the state of the person's thinking when suppression is summoned. As a rule, our thoughts seem to be *stopped* just before we try to suppress. The state of mind that precedes suppression is not the usual rapidly changing stream of consciousness, but rather a single thought or "fixed idea." William James pointed out that normal consciousness contains not just one idea at a time, but rather an assembly of ideas. While we are thinking of one most focally, the "fringes" of past ideas are still evident as they leave, and those of future ideas seem to be forming.[27] When our minds stop on one idea, we have reached what James called an exceptional mental state, a trance of sorts that is clearly a departure from normal consciousness. He remarked that "in a healthy life, there are no single ideas."[28]

The reason thought suppression occurs, then, is simple: *We suppress thoughts that tend to stop our thinking.* When our minds grind to a halt, for any reason, we often invoke suppression as a standard mental repair routine. When we find our minds "fixed" on the idea of a friend's death, for instance, we suppress the thought. Thought "stoppage" seems likely for most every item on the list of most unwanted thoughts we just reviewed. These thoughts are not problems because they are *frequent*, but rather because they are, by some criterion, *too* frequent. We find that we stop to view them more than we would like, and we wish to get our minds moving on to other things once again.

Each of the thoughts people want to suppress acts as an obstacle to further thought. The churchgoer who entertains thoughts of being naked in church, for example, may find the image just too detestable to think, and so stops short just after the thought arrives in his mind. It is probably not the case that the thought occurs very often, and indeed, for a nonreligious person the thought might even be funny and entertaining during a long church service. But the individual who *is* religious can envision the wrath of the clergy, the other parishioners, and even God, not to mention personal guilt, at the event—and thus finds that this thought brings all thinking to a stop. The action must not be done, the emotions must not be felt, and the idea must not even be told. All these prohibitions make the mind lurch. There is nothing left to think at this juncture, and suppression is likely.

Having thought come to a halt is a strange phenomenon. Marvin Minsky, one of the founders of the field of artificial intelligence,[29] has a version of this "stopping" theory based on his observation of computer wackiness. He points out that programmers spend much of their time at the computer not in programming, but in *debugging*, removing logical inconsistencies that keep a program from doing what it is intended to do. The "unwanted thoughts" in programs are bugs, failures in logic that hang up the program and stop it from processing correctly. According to Minsky, ideal programs would include suppression or "censor" subprograms in their instructions to the computer. These censors could reject bugs as they happen in the computation, and thus free the computer to go on computing. The implication for humans, of course, is that we have bugs, too, and that we use mental censors to help us suppress cognitive errors.

Perhaps the most delightful aspect of Minsky's theory is the role he suggests for humor in the human debugging process. Laughing, after all, is a fine way to clear your head. There is nothing like hooting out loud, breathing in great gasps, and drawing your face into a loony grimace to empty the mind. It makes sense that we have an automatic thought-avoidance mechanism that helps us to get rid of thoughts that would otherwise be mental bugs, dead ends, or failures of logic that would leave a simpler computer jammed forever. Humor acts as a restart procedure, a way of beginning a new line of thought when we have reached a mental impasse. This indicates why it is that some of those people faced with the thought of being naked in church, rather than simply trying to stop the thought, might first take a moment to snicker at it.

Most of the things we find funny do have a "wrong-headedness" to them. They indicate wrong actions, improper logic, and minor errors of all kinds. But it is interesting that even the most wrongheaded idea is not likely to be permanently laughable. Jokes are not as funny after the first time or two we've heard them. Minsky explains that jokes wear thin because once we have laughed initially, we have successfully "debugged" that area of thought. We will not be halted or stymied by it again. Of course, some people will laugh repeatedly at the same kinds of things, and this is perhaps because their mental systems have severe difficulties with bugs in certain areas. Their thoughts are easily stopped in those areas, and laughing is one way to clear the slate and start thinking again. Freud may have something to add here, as there certainly do seem to be people who laugh primarily about certain themes—sex, death, bodily functions—perhaps as a result of childhood experiences that left these babies buggy. He wrote extensively about the role of humor in revealing the person's unconscious store of past experiences, and even suggested that what people laugh at might be used to diagnose their problems.[30]

Doing, Saying, and Feeling. Laughter, however, does not always kick in at the right time. There are unwanted thoughts that lead us too quickly to despair, or that somehow short-circuit humor as an automatic debugging strategy. For these thoughts, conscious attempts to suppress become our only resort. When we sit lost in unwanted thoughts as we grieve the death of a loved one, for instance, laughter does not arise automatically to sweep the thoughts away. It probably could not do so, after all, as there are too many reminders of the tragedy at present for us to suppress the thought for more than an instant. But there may be a few laughs mixed with the tears, and eventually the circumstances may become different enough to allow us at least a smile of resignation. Although humor can be a great source of renewal at the right moments, it is not always alone sufficient to help us get on with our thinking.

Getting on with our thinking, however, is crucial. Unwanted thoughts stop us in our mental tracks. They disturb the normal flow of consciousness, bringing it to focus on one or a relatively small number of thoughts. We think about one thing constantly, our intense attention to it punctuated only by our attempts to get away. And with this notion in hand, we can begin now to explore the key topic of this chapter: the circumstances in our lives that lead us to have unwanted thoughts.

Unwanted thoughts are a problem whenever our mind comes to a halt. This happens when it encounters some obstacle to further thinking. The obstacle can be (1) something we don't want to do, (2) something we don't want to say, or (3) something we don't want to feel. In each of these cases, thought precedes something that we wish not to have happen, and so we stop it. Doing, saying, and feeling are all public, irrevocable signs of our thoughts. We advertise what we were just thinking when we eat fudge, call someone a name, or break down crying. Because these signs all make known, for us and for others, what we are thinking, they serve as barriers to further thought. After all, actions, talk, and emotions are all very real consequences of our otherwise hidden thought processes. We hope to stop our thinking when these consequences are on the horizon.

Whenever action, talk, or expression must be avoided, then, our thinking comes to a stop. We must not think of that, we say to ourselves, for fear we will do, say, or show it, and the unwanted thought is formed. Although it may seem that the thought itself is what we don't want, actually it is the consequence of the thought we are concerned about, and the thought blocks our further thinking as a way of avoiding that consequence. With this idea in mind, we can now review some of the thoughts from the "most unwanted" list and see how they came to be that way. The thought of crashing the car on purpose may be a "stopper," for instance, because we have had that thought while driving—and have actually found ourselves fighting to keep from turning the wheel. We stop the thought to stop the act.

The thought of a drink when we are on the wagon is similarly unwanted. It suggests that the next thought should be one of going to get the drink, and this chain must be stopped before we get to the bottle. Again, thought suppression is performed to help in action inhibition. The thought of a loved one dying, on the other hand, is something that normally precedes emotional expression—weeping, perhaps, or at least a shiver of sorrow. To stop the feeling, we stop at the thought and wish it away. The thought of telling someone about a humiliating incident in our past is, likewise, the prelude to an unwanted external state of affairs. We may not want to see the listeners' disapproving looks, or hear the awkward replies, when we reveal the incident to them. So, we stop at the thought, before we say anything, and decide it is the thought we do not want.

We stop our usual chain of associations when we reach certain thoughts to stop the events that may follow. The mental landscape that surrounds us when we stop becomes unwanted, and we try to find new thoughts with which we can ride away from this desolate place in our minds. To see the implications of this, it is important to examine the key consequences of thinking that can make our thoughts unwanted—action, talk, and emotional expression. Action is what we avoid when we attempt *self-control;* talk is what we wish to circumvent when we seek *secrecy;* emotional expression is what we are hoping to stop when we look for *mental peace.* The desires to control ourselves, keep secrets, and keep our minds at peace are common precursors to thought suppression.

Self-Control and Suppression. There are a great many things in life better left undone. And tragically, it is often all too easy to come up with the idea of an act, even when the act itself should never be done. Most people in the modern world know what it would mean to start a nuclear war, for instance. Although we know the label for this action and can even envision "pushing the button," it is something that must never happen. Every act we wish not to do, then, sets up a kind of schism in our minds: We have the thought, but we prefer not to implement it.

The cases when self-control is most clearly responsible for unwanted thoughts are those in which the thoughts are about the obvious goal of the action. Food thoughts in the person on a diet, for instance, are a classic case. When we diet, we become obsessed with food—at least for a while. We begin to agree with Oscar Wilde in *The Picture of Dorian Gray* that "the only way to get rid of a temptation is to yield to it. Resist it, and your soul grows sick with longing for the things it has forbidden to itself."

The case of dieting has been studied by many scientists, and one of the leading current theories of obesity fits our view of unwanted thoughts exactly. This is the *restraint theory*. According to this theory, people who are most inclined to overeat are those who approach food with restraint in mind.[31] One early hint that restraint could cause overeating came from the American conscientious objectors during World War II who agreed to participate in experiments on starvation. When they later began normal diets and returned to their initial weight, they had a persistent tendency to binge at meals, gorging themselves to the maximum of their physical capacity.[32]

People who diet are usually identified in studies of restraint by means of a questionnaire that simply asks how much they try to diet and restrain themselves from eating. Those who identify themselves as "restrainers" on this test approach food in a way that is very unlike "non-restrainers." For example, some of the participants in a study were asked to drink a milkshake at the beginning of the research session[33] They then were told that the study was to examine ice-cream flavor preferences. Each person was given two large bowls to sample. Other people in this study were not given the initial milkshake, but also were asked to sample from two large bowls in the "taste test." The preference between ice creams in the taste test, it turns out, was not really an important part of the study to the experimenters. They were interested instead in how much total ice cream people would eat.

The non-restrainers in this study did what one might think was normal: Those who had their stomachs preloaded by the milkshake sampled much less of the taste-test ice cream than those who had not had the milkshake. This makes sense. They were full, so they stopped. The restrainers, however, followed a different strategy. Those who had no preload milkshake sampled the ice cream very lightly. Those who had already finished the milkshake, in contrast, went on to pig out on the ice cream. The restrainers were able to restrain themselves up to a point—and then lost their composure completely and dove into the food. Ironically, they ate the most when they were already full.

This is strongly reminiscent of the white bear findings. Recall that people who were asked to think about a white bear after they had earlier suppressed the thought became unusually preoccupied with it. In this study, between initial suppression and subsequent preoccupation the experimenter steps in and changes the task—from don't think to think. In the restrainer study, no one had to tell the restrainers when to stop restraining and go for the ice cream. Rather, the preload milkshake served this purpose. Their restraint toward food was destroyed by that preload, and then there was no stopping them. This did not happen among non-restrainers, suggesting that without the initial attempt to suppress thoughts of food, the turnaround to overeating does not follow an initial splurge.

Restrainers are everywhere. With respect to food, more than half the population claims to diet. But there are lots of other attractive things to consume and then try to quit: Alcohol, tobacco, and drugs are the most familiar addictive substances, and their consumption is likely to follow the restraint pattern as well. Once a person is using some addictive substance, he or she is in the same position everyone is with regard to food—it is a regularly experienced pleasure. And once in this position, we can restrain or not. Quitting, of course, is the ultimate restraint, and it is just at this time that the recurrence of unwanted thought leaps up to surprise us.

Quitting can lead to an obsession, at least temporarily.[34] Although *during* our addiction, we may have thought about our particular habit infrequently, perhaps before each use, once we try to quit we become obsessed with it. Now, there are reasons to become obsessed that are certainly unrelated to our difficulty in dealing with unwanted thoughts. In the case of tobacco, alcohol, and many drugs, our bodies develop physiological dependencies that remind us, like hunger, of the addictive substances we desire. This alone is often enough to draw our attention. But in these cases, it is likely that an additional burden is always added to physical cravings by the very fact of our self-control.

The more we try to control our thoughts, the more inclined we are to suffer a relapse to addiction. Clinical psychologists who study how people fall back on addictive substances suggest there is an *abstinence relapse* phenomenon, a tendency to think about the habit more after a failure in abstinence than during a period of uninterrupted use.[35] The smoker who has just one cigarette after going cold turkey, for example, often seems to quit quitting with a vengeance, and relapses to high levels of tobacco use. Alcoholics, too, find just one drink can be their downfall. And with heroin, cocaine, or tranquilizers, it may require only one relapse after abstinence to bring back the habit at full force.

In these cases, it seems that traversing the thin line from suppression to obsession takes only a single step. People do not seem to follow a period of successful suppression with a "sample and quit again" approach. Although this can be done, the more common pattern is for one fall off the wagon to leave the person lying in the ditch. Although it is not yet clear to what degree thought suppression is implicated in these cases, the parallel between these phenomena and the white bear effect is striking. Stopping seems to be hard, but it also makes starting up again dangerously easy.

Self-control can extend beyond food and addictive substances to any behavior at all. Staying with someone who is abusive, for example, seems much like an addiction. We may wish to control our tendency to be around a person who harms us, and so try to break off a relationship. Likewise, nervous habits such as fingernail biting or hair tossing can come under the control umbrella as well. The ballplayer who occasionally throws a wild ball may, too, find this is something worthy of suppression. Anything we do that we do not want to do can start this process. We try not to think of it, and for a while we succeed. But later if we give it just the tiniest quarter in our minds, perhaps by doing it once or starting on the way to do it, the unwanted behavior comes back completely, sometimes with even more energy than before.

Finally, there are some behaviors we wish to control that we have never done before. Like starting the nuclear war, behaviors such as committing suicide or becoming violent enough to kill are ones we try never to do. It may be that in these cases we can still build up powerful preoccupations with the behaviors because we try not to think of them, succeed, and lose track of the whole project, only to be reminded of the problem by some stray thought. The flood of thinking that arrives on the heels of our suppression gets us worried again that we might do the unwanted thing and starts the cycle over again.

When we think of things we are trying not to do, our mind comes to a stop. The lurch we feel when we are so rudely halted gets our attention, and so we try to banish the thought. It is not that thinking about an action *always* causes the action, of course, but it is somewhat troublesome not to slip once in a while and start toward the action if we are thinking about it all the time. So we suppress the thought and, in so doing, we seem to set in motion a process that makes us acutely sensitive to the very thing we are attempting to control. As Dewey observed, "The hard drinker who keeps thinking of not drinking is doing what he can to initiate the acts which lead to drinking. He is starting with the stimulus to his habit."[36] All of this attention and effort can be enough to propagate a flood of thoughts about the target of our self-control, an outpouring that happens if we ever give ourselves the luxury of releasing the suppression.

Secrecy and Suppression. Holding something inside can have the same effect. To recall Oscar Wilde in *The Picture of*

Dorian Gray again: "I have grown to love secrecy. It seems to be the one thing that can make modern life mysterious and marvelous to us. The commonest thing is delightful if only one hides it." When we first decide to keep a secret, we attach a mental reminder to the secret information, and this makes it special. This reminder says that we should not reveal the information if it comes to mind, and probably also contains a list of whom we can tell and whom we can't. The next time we talk to someone who should not know the secret, then, this planned deception is somewhere in the corner of our mind. It may be a plan to deceive by omission, to lie by leaving out some piece of information; it may be a plan to deceive by commission, to lie by fabricating new information that is false.[37]

Secrets are sometimes acts of commission, and in this case we must actively deal with the problem. We must fabricate something from thin air to fill in the space where the truth cannot be said. There is the danger we will bring it up too soon, have the wrong facial expression, react incorrectly when the audience responds to what we say, and so on. In other words, this is a precarious situation and we will have to suppress thinking about the truth the whole time to make sure nothing inappropriate slips out. At least in this case, though, we will have something to think about: the new "facts" we made up to fill in. We will have a focus for our thinking that allows us to concentrate our attention.

When we deceive by omission, there is nothing at all to say or think. We may be lucky, of course, and it may not even come to mind as we talk. But more likely, we will be reminded of the secret by the presence of the person we are trying not to tell. After all, this person is listed as one who shouldn't know, and so will help us recall the secret thought. Or, if we are not reminded even then, and instead just happen to think of the secret thought in the presence of the person, we will have the thought "red-flagged" in our mind. It will be on the tip of our tongue, seemingly ever-ready as the "next thing to say," and always thought of prior to other thoughts we then verbalize as replacements.

When the person we kept the secret from goes away, we can then stop suppressing. We heave a mental sigh of relief and sit back. But now, of course, we are even more inclined to think of our secret next time we see this person. The mental wrestling match we've just finished has made us form an image of the person that now features the secret thought. It is a full-blown "What if he or she knew?" scenario, and this provides a powerful reminder of the thought each time the person comes around. Say, one afternoon at work you and some friends make fun of an overweight co-worker by calling her a tubster behind her back. You will probably remember this every time you see her, mainly because you can't tell her about it.

A thought that is suppressed for social reasons can also be subject to periods of increased and decreased attempted suppression. The presence or absence of the people who are to be left out of the secret serves to turn suppression on or off, and these cyclic turns may have the effect of creating yet further preoccupation with the thought. You can't say "tubster" when she's around, but you all call her the tubster when she's not there. As in the case of the abstinence/relapse cycle of self-control, deception and relaxation of the deception can promote an unstable mental state, one that oscillates between trying not to think and thinking a lot. Each new time you try not to think of the secret, it is again difficult because you have become absorbed with it as a result of the *prior* attempt to suppress it.

Suppose one has a general secret, something one wants to keep from many people, perhaps everyone. I was in this position a while back when my wife and I took it into our heads that we would keep her pregnancy secret for the first couple of months. I'm not sure whether we were more concerned about how people at her workplace would respond, or about waiting until the early dangers of miscarriage were over. In either case, we hoped to do this for just a few weeks, or until further deception required the use of a portable plywood enclosure. On seeing people the first day after we had made the pact, each of us wanted to spill the beans. I had to try dearly not to talk or think about it in the presence of every audience I encountered.

The secret is big news, however, and thus tends to come to mind as the first thing one wants to say in meeting a friend. "What's new?" they ask. The answer to this question is ready, but I'm not able. Unfortunately, one does not usually keep a second-in-line thought for the purpose of immediate disclosure in this situation. So, I am at a loss. I say that nothing is new, and even though I recall real news (other than the secret) at a later point, it just doesn't jump forward the way it should. Somehow, withholding the most important thought keeps everything back a bit, so I end up revealing nothing but obvious thoughts, observations on the weather, and the like. I become more boring than I want to be.

On getting used to suppression with that first audience, one eventually comes out of one's shell and engages again in conversation. Sometimes I even forgot completely that I had a secret—until I saw another person I knew. Then, it came right back—for, after all, I had to remember not to mention it to *this* person as well. Each new friend I encountered, especially the close ones I usually tell most everything, brought back the thought and made me renew the resolve to suppress it and avoid talking. Several days went by, and I became progressively more practiced in suppression, actually forgetting for hours and hours that I had something to hide. But all it took was an encounter with someone I hadn't met since we'd acquired our secret, and the suppression experience returned.

Eventually, we did tell. And a wonderful baby was born who is certainly no secret any longer. There are some secrets, however, that can last a lifetime. We may have traumas or dilemmas that we attempt to cover up and pretend never happened. All the things that society thinks are improper or tragic, of course, one will not want to reveal. This includes things we may do on purpose that hurt people or break moral rules: We keep secret our crimes, our manipulations of others, our scandalous sexual activities, and even our desires to do these things. But we may also avoid revealing many things over which we had no control, the points in life when we were victimized: We keep secret the times we were fooled, seduced, humiliated, hurt, molested, or abandoned.

We avoid public display of these kinds of incidents because we know that we might be stigmatized by them. We know of people who have been marked in one way or another by their lives, and we hope to avoid the consequences, real or imagined, of being in some way infamous.[38] But in the rush to avoid social disapproval, we take the conflict into our own heads. Rather than being social pariahs ourselves, we allow certain of our thoughts to become stigmatized in our minds. We reject them once, and then again and again. And, as in the case of many unwanted thoughts, they may finally run our lives.

In a series of striking observations, James Pennebaker has shown the toll that secrets can take.[39] In one study, many of the people responding to a national magazine poll who reported frequent health problems were found to have something to hide. More of these people than would be expected had been abused or sexually molested as children. Follow-up surveys conducted with other participants showed that health problems seemed to ensue only when people who were traumatized early in life failed to tell others of their experience. The studies indicate that victims of traumas who do reveal their thoughts and feelings to others tend to feel awful during the confession—but show measurable improvements in immune function and general health, as well as reduced physiological signs of stress, in the months that follow.

In trying not to talk, and so keep a secret to ourselves, we freeze our thoughts in place. The thought of the secret sticks in our mind as a way of making the secret stick in our throat, and we come to the same mental impasse we find in every case of unwanted thoughts. We cannot think beyond our current thought because we are afraid of what would happen if we did.

Mental Peace and Suppression. Some thoughts lead to painful emotional expression. Whenever we think of dying, for example, we can soon get choked up in self-pity and despair. Does it all have to end so soon? Who will take care of the house pets? The thought of death can bring on a tearful interlude, perhaps even an intense depression, and so we find that this thought often blocks further thinking whenever it occurs. Dwelling on this would produce emotions we hope to avoid. The thoughts that produce strong emotions are especially fitting candidates for suppression.

Many people lead remarkably unemotional lives because they exercise mental control to keep the emotions from happening. Freud remarked on the common repression of emotions in certain psychological disorders, and clinical psychologists since have often recommended emotional expression or "catharsis" as a way of overcoming psychological problems.[40] At the extreme, there are even therapists who believe people can benefit by going into a room on a regular basis and screaming themselves hoarse. Looking at this from the viewpoint of mental control, however, we can see that such outpourings of emotion are probably poor cures for anything. The only emotions that we really need to express are those that are blocking our thinking. Certain very specific emotions may be preventing mental peace, and they may not involve screaming at all.

These unwanted emotions may not even be that negative. The pursuit of mental peace is the avoidance of *unwanted* emotional states, not negative ones. Normally, we suppress thoughts that could lead us to negative emotions, as these are the feelings we do not want to have. It is conceivable, however, that we might also wish to avoid the expression of positive emotions under some circumstances. There are times when we seem satisfied to dwell on the darker side, sing the blues, and wallow in the most vile thoughts we can imagine. Horror films are one instance of such attraction. Or we may hope to avoid laughing during an argument because we wish to stay mad for a while longer. These observations suggest that the particular content of an emotion is not, by itself, sufficient for us to suppress the thought that precedes it. Just because a thought is likely to lead us to a negative emotion does not mean we will necessarily stop thinking when it comes.

Rather, thought suppression must come from the *relation* between a thought and one's emotional state of mind. A thought thus may be suppressed when it is in conflict with other thoughts. As a rule, we are in a positive or at least a neutral mood, thinking well of ourselves and our worlds. So, for the most part, it is negative emotions we will avoid. Thus, we may normally be in a frame of mind that makes us want to avoid an unhappy thought or suppress a disgusting image. But on occasion we find we are in a generally negative mental state. When this happens, we may find ourselves avoiding positive thoughts because of the positive emotions that they may evoke. Here, we may avoid a happy memory just because it conflicts with our gloomy frame of mind.

A complication in all this comes when we realize that mental turmoil can itself produce emotion. As we have noted, mental peace departs when our thoughts stop to prevent some unwanted emotion. It may even be the case, however, that we develop unwanted emotions from the very occurrence of repetitive thoughts themselves. We find we are thinking something too often, and this observation makes us not want to think it the next time. If we did think it, we might then experience the alarm that comes when we believe our mind cannot be controlled. The emotions that come from lack of mental control—fear of racing thoughts, anxiety about uncontrollable mental states, a mood of desperation—can in this way feed back to yield suppression. The desire not to show how disturbed we are by our own chain of thinking, in short, can cause us to bring our thoughts to a stop. And then, all that is left is the desire to put the unwanted thought out of mind.

Mental peace, like self-control and secrecy, is a goal that can be far more elusive than we imagine. It turns out that trying not to feel, like trying not to behave or to talk, can throw a monkey wrench into our mental apparatus. We stop at the thought that precedes any of these unwanted effects of thinking, and in this way we reach a true "mental block." The only way around it is to suppress the thought, and even when we do this, the suppressed thought can return and stop our thinking again and again. Thought suppression comes from trying to keep thoughts from escaping our mind and affecting what we do, say, and feel. When we keep them prisoner in this way, though, we shouldn't then be surprised when they will not go away.

With these ideas in place about why we suppress thoughts, we can now begin to consider how we do it. The suppression of a thought, of course, depends on the occurrence of a thought, so we need to understand something about how thought occurs. We must dismantle a thinking machine and see how it operates. In the next chapter, we use this tactic of learning by destruction—the same one children favor whenever they are curious about expensive toys—to look into the human mental apparatus.

THREE

The Mental Apparatus

*The human being is a machine. An automatic machine. It is
composed of thousands of complex and delicate mechanisms,
which perform their functions harmoniously and perfectly,
in accordance with laws devised for their governance
and over which the man himself has no authority,
no mastership, no control.*

—Mark Twain, *Letters from the Earth*

Just because we have minds doesn't mean we know how
to operate them. Imagine, for instance, getting a new microwave
oven, taking it out of the box, and plugging it in, but not finding
the instructions. For your first meal, you incinerate a chicken
pot pie. For your next, you vulcanize a hot dog. The third time
you manage to boil water successfully, so you enjoy a nice big
cup of hot water. This is precisely the position we are in with
our mind—hot water. We get this marvelous high-tech machine
on our birthday, and there are no instructions to be found.

We spend our whole lives, then, trying to figure out how our
mind works. This wonderful contraption has some capacities
we never discover; it has other abilities we learn about and use
repeatedly; it has yet other tricks we know about but can't make
happen when we want them. In this chapter, we will consider
the mind as though it were a machine—a viewpoint taken by
some cognitive scientists and students of artificial intelligence.[41]
We will explore what sort of machine it is, and investigate how
it is that such a machine has the extraordinary property of *trying*

to control itself. Unlike the microwave oven, the mind cooks up its own instructions over time, learning how to operate itself. It develops preferences about its own modes of operation, coming to hold some thoughts as wanted and others as unwanted. What kind of mental apparatus is necessary for this to happen?

Artificial Insanity.   It is consoling to know, right off the bat, that computers suffer from the same problems we do. Their mental apparatus can have difficulties that very much resemble our struggles with unwanted thoughts. We have all seen it. Science fiction movies show us computers gone awry, their banks of lights flashing urgently while printouts sail into tangles, tapes unreel, and showers of sparks illuminate the room. The obvious fix-up in these cases, of course, is to pull the plug, and this usually seems to restore calm in short order. Something vaguely like this does occur in real life, and anyone who has operated a personal computer or word processor knows that the machine can reach unwanted states at times.

Computers can get caught in their own internal logic, sometimes going out of control, and sometimes just shutting down so that their operators can't get a message in through the keyboard. And, just as in the movies, these true computer "nervous breakdowns" can usually be fixed by turning the machine off and on again. This happened to me once when I was trying to teach myself the BASIC programming language. Having read the manual for well over a minute, I sat down at the computer to take a first spin. The manual suggested beginning with a PRINT command, just an instruction to the machine to print on the screen something I had told it to print. The manual also suggested making this first statement be "I am a computer programmer." In a more humble mood than this, I began by trying to print "Back to basics."

The book said to type in an instruction (PRINT "Back to basics"), and then to type the word RUN. I wasn't entirely clear on what this was all about, but I typed a facsimile anyway and typed RUN to see it work. The first time I typed RUN, nothing happened, so I tried it again. The phrase "Back to basics" appeared on every line of the screen, and the keyboard locked up so that I could no longer control the process at all.

I had to reset the machine—turn it off and on again—and on looking over the program, I found the problem. The word RUN, which normally is a signal to follow the commands in a program that stands outside the program, had been embedded here in the program itself. The way I had done things made the program contain two lines of instruction to the computer—my PRINT line and another line saying RUN. Thus, the program started by PRINTing my little phrase, and then executed a command to RUN, and so began itself again. The RUN command was not only *in* the program but also was *about* the program, and so produced an infinite loop that my PC could not stop executing. There is something about this that seems highly relevant to the white bear problem. Just like the human who can't stop thinking of an unwanted thought, the computer here seemed obsessed with a thought of its own.

It turns out that computer programmers use procedures based on exactly this trick all the time. Computer programs commonly have the ability to follow instructions that are *about* the instructions. This capacity is called *recursion*, and it was an example of this that I stumbled upon in making my first little BASIC program. Recursive functions often occur in a loop, a portion of the program that is designed to repeat itself. But it does not usually repeat itself exactly. It changes itself as it repeats, thus creating *new* instructions as it carries on. This ability is extremely valuable in programming, as it allows for progressive change in the program. Anyone who has pro-grammed will soon find, however, that it is very easy to incorporate unwanted loops in programs. Recursion must be used, but it carries with it the continued danger of program processes that will repeat themselves infinitely or otherwise get wildly out of hand.

The human mental apparatus does not allow the same "save" that computer operaters hold dear: We have no handy reset button on the back of our head. But we do have some interesting controls anyway. Unlike computers, we seem capable often of "stepping outside" repeating mental processes, while remaining in our own head. Even if we cannot control loops immediately, we can tell that they have become faulty or cyclic, and we thus can set out to control ourself. Very few of us, after all, would type "Back to basics" forever.[42] We notice that we are thinking again and again about an incident that made us jealous of our mate, for example, but instead of repeating the thought forever we may soon do something to fix it. The "repair" may be a heart-to-heart talk, a decision to get closer to our mate, or perhaps a decision to do something that will make us more distant so the jealousy is not so bothersome. This suggests that our mental apparatus is considerably more sophisticated than the wiring of a personal computer, somehow fixing itself even when it reaches a severe impasse.

To understand how these observations apply to the problem of unwanted thoughts, it is important to examine the mental apparatus in some detail. Can human thought be described in the same way we describe computer programs? Can we speak of *mental* loops like those in a computer program? If so, what would the loop look like that is responsible for our problems in suppressing the thought of a white bear? Addressing these kinds of questions requires setting computers aside and concentrating directly on people.

Cognition and Metacognition. An important starting point for examining the mental apparatus is the realization that people not only think, but think about their thinking. The term *cognition* refers to thinking; *metacognition* is the term for thoughts about thinking. Loosely speaking, the process of thinking is something people do to things inside their head. This definition highlights the most obvious quality of thought—its character of having an object. We think about things, and the curious quality of thought is that it requires something to be *about*. It is clear that when we muse on the neighbor's yappy dog, for example, or review what happened the time the neighbor stepped on a rake, we are thinking, for we have these objects to consider. When our mind has no object, it is difficult to argue that thought is going on.

Metacognition occurs when thought takes itself as an object. Imagine you are on a diet, and you keep thinking about having a chocolate. When you decide you would rather not think about chocolate, you are engaging in metacognition. Your metacognitive activity need not settle on any single thought, however, as it can extend to many different thoughts as a group (such as all foods, everything in the kitchen, or—as in the case of my tragic diets—all further pleasure until the end of time). For that matter, your metacognitions may even be about your thought processes and capacities. The fact is, you can think about your inability to avoid chocolate thoughts, about what might be a good strategy for making yourself avoid them, or even about what usually sets them off. These ideas about how your mind works are thoughts about processes of thinking, and so qualify as metacognitions.

Metacognition lies at the very heart of mental control. To control our own mind, we must think about it, grasp what it is doing, and exert some form of influence on its course of action. The first step in this sequence would seem to be simply thinking about our thoughts—in other words, engaging in metacognition. To desire thinking about a warm summer evening at the ocean (while we are not doing so), or likewise, to fear thinking of an ugly scene from a horror film (while we are not doing so), we must be able to think about potential thoughts. This is not all we need to do, of course, because just knowing about something is not the same as controlling it. Knowing we are going to "go blank" when we get up to talk in front of a crowd, for instance, is not the same as stopping ourself from going blank. But metacognition is a first step, a giant step. It is something we can do that microwave ovens cannot.

There is a resemblance, however, between our capacity for metacognition and the computer's capacity for recursion. Recall that silly program I wrote that had one line calling for the machine to PRINT and another calling for the program to RUN. In a way, the PRINT statement is like a simple thought or cognition, whereas the RUN statement is like a metacognition. The PRINT statement was in the program, as was the RUN statement. But the RUN statement was also *about* the program— it was an instruction to the computer to carry out the program (which contained both PRINT and RUN). The analogy is an interesting one because it suggests that there is something potentially dangerous about metacognition. Like the RUN statement in the program, metacognition might just be the culprit behind human problems with repeating thoughts.

The RUN statement in the program, like many metacognitions, has the unusual property of *self-reference*. It is about itself. The sentence "This sentence is false" is about itself in this way, and when we try to understand what it means we quickly arrive at a paradox.[43] You see, if the sentence is false, then it is false that "This sentence is false," so the sentence is true—and if it is true, then it is true that "This sentence is false," so it is false. The self-referent quality of the sentence makes its interpretation problematic in a very special way. There is something about things that refer to themselves that wreaks havoc with our sense of what is logical and right. And though this is often the case, we should note, however, that this puzzling quality is not inevitable. The sentence "This sentence is true," for instance, isn't all that paradoxical. It is just sort of stupid. It could sit there being true until the end of time, and never really matter at all.

The Logic of Metacognition. To understand the quirky, perplexing aspect of metacognition, we must take a closer look at the "meta" idea in general. A good place to begin is with Russell's paradox, a mathematical problem that lies at the center of this idea. Like me, you may assume that balancing the checkbook is the only math problem really worth solving. Mathematicians, however, point out that the checkbook balancing is trivial once we have solved a more fundamental question: Can a class be a member of itself? I know this doesn't sound as if it will affect the monthly balance, but mathematicians insist it will. This is because much of the theory of mathematics is based on the idea that numbers can be grouped together into classes (such as all odd numbers, all numbers between 0 and 10, or all positive checking balances), and the question of whether a class can "belong" to itself seems to arise frequently. After all, sometimes it seems perfectly reasonable for a class to be a member of itself. If we consider the class of "everything," for example, it seems sensible to argue that this general class of "everything," just like any particular member of this class, is *some*thing, and therefore belongs to the class of "everything." By this logic, "everything" can be a member of the class of "everything."

Early in this century, the logician Gottlob Frege was just finishing the second volume of his life work, *The Fundamentals of Arithmetic,* when he received a letter from Bertrand Russell. Frege had based his theory of mathematics on the assumption that a set could be a member of itself, but Russell's letter pointed out that this assumption yielded a paradox—a contradiction that entirely undermined Frege's theory. The theory was about to be published, so all Frege could do was insert a footnote on Russell's point, one that sounded much like "never mind my life work." Later on, Russell and Whitehead published *Principia Mathematica,* a theory that circumvented the paradox and, in so doing, made way for an important point about the nature of metacognition.[44]

We can start to see the rub that Russell did when we observe that most classes are not members of themselves. The class of "shrubbery," for example, is not itself a shrub. This means some classes might be members of themselves and some might not. Russell grasped this distinction to produce his paradox: If we consider the class of all those classes that are not members of themselves, the question arises if this grand class is a member of itself. If it is, then it belongs to the class of all those classes that are not members of themselves, and like those classes has the property of not being a member of itself—and so is not. If it is not, however, then it does not belong to the class of all those classes that are not members of themselves, and thus cannot share with them the property of not being a member of itself—and so it is. To shorten the logic, it appears that if it is, it isn't, and if it isn't, it is. A contradiction ensues when we allow a class to be a member of itself.

Russell's solution to this paradox was to legislate it out of existence. He simply held that classes could not be members of themselves, and that was that. Mathematicians continue to argue about the elegance of this solution, and even Russell called the theory "inchoate, confused, and obscure."[45] The proposal was that the mixture of a class and its members in the same statement constitutes a "confusion of types." In this view, members and classes are different logical types, and speaking of both in a way that is not reducible to either one alone produces a line of thinking that typically leads to paradoxes of the form of the class/member paradox. (This includes the "barber paradox"—the barber who shaves all those men in town, and only those men, who do not shave themselves. Who shaves the barber?)

To see the psychological parallel to this, we need to recognize that thoughts *about* thoughts have a relationship that logically parallels the relationship between classes and members. Just as class must be distinguished from member, a thought about a thought must be distinguished from the thought that it is about; the first is of a different logical type than the second.[46] This distinction has been made not just for thoughts, but for forms of language in general by the Polish mathematician Alfred Tarski.[47] His idea was to give names to Russell's logical types. According to his conventions, statements about the world are usually said in "object language," whereas statements about these statements are expressed in "metalanguage."

To say "Elephants are our friends," for example, is a statement in object language. To comment on the truth or falsity of this statement, or just to say that the statement is goofy, must be said in metalanguage. Of course, there are not only two levels to this system. If someone said, "Calling 'Elephants are our friends' a goofy statement is a cruel thing to say," this person would be talking in meta-metalanguage. There can thus be multiple levels of metalanguage. Each level is defined relatively, however, in that the lower-level language can be treated as an object language for the higher-level metalanguage.

When we apply these ideas to thinking, important questions arise. Is the basic fabric of thought only a single "level" of internal language, an object language of sorts, or does it contain additional levels, higher-order sets of thoughts that refer to the lower levels? And if we admit to such levels in thinking, then how many should we have? Clearly, as Russell has noted, even two levels are trouble when they are linked in an interdependent way. The notion that people can think about their thoughts brings with it the immediate and seemingly cataclysmic possibility of an infinite mental regress. If we can metathink about a thought, what is to keep us from meta-metathinking about metathoughts, and so on, until we think at infinite levels about finite thoughts?

We can see a solution to this problem, and at the same time develop a basic picture of the mental apparatus, with one observation. As Tarski pointed out, metalanguage statements always say something about the degree to which the object-level statement should or should not be in the class of object-level statements. They comment on the truth or falsity, goodness or badness, acceptance or rejection, wantedness or unwantedness, of statements at the object level. Nothing "new" can be added at the meta level that is not directly *about* an object-level statement. So, when we say "I would rather not think about the divorce," for instance, we are rejecting at the meta level all "divorce thoughts" at the object level. Or, when we say "I think you are telling the truth," we are using metalanguage to welcome a thought ("what you said") into the object-language world.

This means that all metacognition can be viewed as the relative emphasis or deemphasis of object-level thoughts. There may be colorations of object-level thoughts that are produced at the meta level ("Saying 'Elephants are our friends' is wonderfully insightful"), but the impact of these at the object level is always merely to affirm or deny the object-level thought. And even a high-level monstrosity such as a meta-meta-meta-metathought is really only a paper tiger when it is viewed in this way. At each higher level, some comment is being made about what should or shouldn't be present at the level just below. So, each new level we add at the top has only the effect of producing relative *shadings* of the level just below it, and this transformation happens over and over all the way down to the object level.

All metacognition, in this analysis, can be reduced to two simple forms—the emphasis and deemphasis of thoughts. No matter how high we climb on the ladder of thinking about thinking about thinking about thinking . . . , the result is only a relative concentration on certain object-level thoughts or a relative suppression of certain object-level thoughts. This means that the mind can be represented quite well as an apparatus with only two levels, the object level and a single level of metacognition. All possible metacognitive statements can be summarized at one level, as they all impinge eventually only on one kind of influence: At the metacognitive level, the mind registers what is okay, or not okay, at the object level. Metacognitions are preferences for our minds, wishes about what we might think.

The Window of Consciousness. So far, we have envisioned a mental apparatus that has two basic parts: a big box of thoughts, and another box that contains the metathoughts (each of which refers to one or more of the thoughts). Obviously, there will need to be more. One crying need, for instance, is for some way to sort through these things and think just one at a time. Otherwise, we are in danger of thinking all our thoughts at once and then having nothing to think for the weekend. The mental apparatus must contain some sort of sweet spot, a little box that holds one thought at a time, the thought we are "thinking."

Psychologists have called this little box "consciousness," "focal attention," "working memory," and lots of other things, but the basic idea is always the same. There has to be a place in the apparatus for what is happening now. Moreover, this spot appears to be relatively small. In a classic article published in 1956, George Miller suggested that the capacity of conscious attention is about seven plus or minus two chunks of information.[48] When we try to remember a phone number between the directory and the phone, for instance, we have trouble if the number is longer than seven plus or minus two digits. This is particularly true if the digits are random and not easily put together in our mind into groups, what Miller called "chunks." We may thus be able to recall a very long number such as 123456789123456789123456789 quite easily. But that is because we don't need to hold random digits in mind, only the well-learned chunk of 123456789 and the additional chunk of three repeats.

The point of this is that consciousness, that fleeting window in our mind from which we view all of our experiences in sequence, is limited. We may feel that we are conscious of many things at the same time, but the number of individual pieces of information we can carry in our conscious mind is not large. The conscious window is thus a proportionately tiny spot in our mind as a whole. The great question of interest, then, is how this tiny spot interacts with the rest of our thoughts. How do things get into the conscious window, what do they do when they're there, and how do they get out?

Certainly, we can observe that both object-level thoughts and metathoughts gain entry to consciousness from time to time. Therefore, there must be some system that makes their travel arrangements. One current guess about how this system works is a simple "association" or "network" model.[49] Such a system leads consciousness from one thought to the next by virtue of associative links; we think "eggs" when we hear "ham" because the two are linked in our memories. We may another time think "pork" or "Hamilton" or even "sausage links" if these things are also linked to "ham" in our memories, but we usually think first of those things that are most strongly linked to a thought, taking more distant associative pathways only if there is a context of other thoughts that leads us in such directions.

This system for conscious thinking allows different thoughts to be brought to mind through a process of "spreading activation." It is as though all our thoughts were a large crowd of people, say at a department store, and consciousness were a mad pincher running through the crowd. Right after the fat man in the umbrellas yelled, we would expect squawks from other people nearby. It would be odd indeed to hear a shriek from sporting goods or a commotion in toys, but we could well expect a tweak in scarves or hats—right down the aisle from the umbrella section. This model of conscious thinking, in short, depends on the idea that certain thoughts are near each other while other thoughts are far apart. The mind travels only by short hops.

Consciousness can embrace any of our potential thoughts, and also any of our metathoughts. Normally, it moves among these various thoughts in its automatic mode. So, when it is in the cheese dip section of our mind, it thinks in turn about things related to dip—chips, crackers, parties, and so on. Eventually, of course, this automatic chain of thinking can move quite far from any starting point. From dips and parties, we might go to the particular party at which Fred skinned his forehead break-dancing on gravel, and this is pretty far from cheese dip (or maybe not). At any rate, the mental apparatus uses consciousness as a moving window that browses through everything we know and perceive, one thing at a time, in a chain of automatic associations. Consciousness does not necessarily know *why* the particular automatic links arise, as it contains just the ideas that are reached and not maps to all of their origins.[50]

One other characteristic of this conscious window deserves note. The conscious window contains information that is most relevant to *what one is doing now*.[51] It typically contains a plan for the dominant action of the moment, and it keeps the person focused on one major thing at a time. So, it ensures that one is ready to do at least one thing at all times during its operation. This is handy. Otherwise, we might be too scattered ever to do anything, and we would have to get jobs with the government.

Automatic and Controlled Thinking. Sometimes thinking feels effortful and sometimes it doesn't. We have already had an introduction to this idea by William James, but now it is time to include this distinction in our model of the mental apparatus. First off, we can point out that automatic forms of thinking seem to occur both inside the conscious window and outside it. Although we can travel through a chain of automatic associations as we watch, it is also possible to do automatic thinking without watching. We can make inferences, be influenced by memories, or even perceive things without knowing we are doing so.[52]

Research on automatic thought indicates that we do a great deal of thinking of which we are only dimly aware. As a rule, for example, we remember about how many times we have seen something before—without ever consciously counting the occurrences. We also tend to remember spatial location information—where something was in a room, on a page, or the like—without attending to this in a controlled way. And we can usually recall temporal information—how long something took, or in what order things happened—without conscious attention either. When we try to do these things on purpose, we don't do them much better than if we don't try at all, so such thought processes appear to occur automatically.[53]

Thinking on purpose, on the other hand, helps certain of our thought processes dramatically. These processes always require consciousness. There is the strong feeling of effort when we work to control our minds, when we devote much attention to what we are doing. Controlled thinking occurs when we try hard to remember, to perceive, or to solve a problem. The principal characteristic of controlled thinking—at least in the way psychologists study it—is that it can be disrupted when additional demands are made on our attention: It takes controlled thinking for people to do long division, for example, because we can demonstrate that when they are distracted by shouts or tickling, they come out with six different answers in a row. Other kinds of thinking do not require so much cognitive capacity, and these we can do with our attention tied behind our back. Perceiving our own name being spoken, for instance, is often automatic even when there are other conversations and noises going on.

Where does metacognition lie on the automatic-controlled dimension? When we do automatic thinking, it seems much of what we do can be described as following links between object-level thoughts. Thus, for example, when you have a chain of thoughts, or even a repeating cycle that doesn't seem to stop, you may be experiencing an automatic process. Thoughts of "Saturday" lead to thoughts of "family reunion" which lead to thoughts of "finding the potato salad recipe" and on and on . . . in a chain that skips along automatically. Some automatic associations, however, are between object-level thoughts and metathoughts. We may move immediately, for example, from the thought of "blood" to a metathought like "I'd rather not think of this, thanks." It doesn't take any great effort to be revolted and leap to this conclusion. The translation from the meta level back to the object level, however, is not so automatic. In fact, this is the point at which automatic thinking commonly gives way to conscious and effortful mental control.

Metathoughts don't just move us instantaneously toward or away from the object thoughts to which they refer. Rather, they serve as guideposts on the road and make us do the movements ourselves. So, for instance, to avoid the thought of blood may require a fancy mental dodge. We might need to move from one metathought to another, translating "I don't want to think about blood" to "I think I'll review the organization of my underwear drawer." Although it is certainly possible that our attempts at mental control could become well learned and habitual, and so fly by in an automatic way, it seems most often the case that we must work to change our conscious thinking. It takes most of our attention to influence our conscious window.

This is why metathoughts can seem to succeed or fail, whereas object-level thoughts do not have these properties. When you think of that attractive person of the noticeably opposite sex you saw on the beach, for instance, you just are thinking and that's all. There is no question of whether such an object-level thought "succeeds" or "fails," because it just "happens" to you. When you have a metathought, of course, it also "happens"— the impulse to daydream about that beach scene may drop in automatically from the blue as well. But when you attempt to implement a metathought, it can very well not work. When the dentist is drilling in your mouth and you are trying desperately to enact a metathought ("Concentrate on the beach, quick"), it may fail. Metathoughts are instructions we give ourselves about our object-level thinking, and sometimes we just can't follow our own instructions.

In essence, metathoughts are instructions for the conscious window to *change its own contents*. This odd sort of transformation takes special care, extra attention, and at least for a while, a conscious concern with what is in consciousness itself.

Every time we start monkeying with what is in our conscious-ness—or what will be in it shortly—we are using controlled thinking to attempt to implement a metacognition. Controlled thought, unlike the automatic variety, is directed by a conscious goal. We want to know the answer to a long-division problem, so we keep working it through until the answer appears; we want to see what everyone is pointing toward in the distance, so we keep looking until we find out; we want to avoid thinking of a white bear, so we keep working on thinking of other things until the white bear goes away.

During all this, automatic thought processes keep chugging along—performing the simple parts of the long-division calcu-lations, directing our eyes and sorting the patterns we see when we look in the distance, and guiding the associations we make to distract ourselves from the white bear. Automatic thought carries on the background operations of our minds, only on occasion to be directed or disturbed by metacognitions. When metacognitions do step in, they do not operate automatically. Instead, they must lumber into the light of the conscious window to try to change the view. As it turns out, this is a key part of their inability to succeed in the immediate suppression of a thought.

We have noted that the conscious window is somewhat lim-ited, in that it holds the thoughts that are happening *now*. Many other thought processes must also occur now, in the present, for this is the only time when anything at all can actually happen. The past is over, and the future is not yet. This much we know from Dickens's *A Christmas Carol*. But more to the point, it appears that many automatic thought processes can occur now, at once, because they do not have to squeeze into the conscious window to get their work done. These processes carry on *parallel* to one another in time. They can be uninformed about each other and uncoordinated as well, but still complete their simple little jobs. This is what allows us to walk, listen to music, chew gum, talk about the weather, and look at a passing car at the same time. These things are largely automatic and run separate, parallel courses.

Conscious thoughts, in contrast, follow one another in a roughly *serial* pattern over time. Each one comes into consciousness for its brief moment in the light, it does its work or at least tries to, and then it is shoved away by the next thought in line. Miller's number of thoughts (seven plus or minus two) are the most we can get into our conscious window at once. Our difficult time with thought suppression comes when, in this sequence of conscious thoughts, we get the idea to *suppress a current thought*. The suppression metathought ("I'd rather not think of a white bear") is here, but the thought ("white bear") is here, too. As long as we continue to hold the metathought in the conscious window, the thought will be there. The thought and metathought do not run in parallel like automatic thoughts, but rather arrive together in their shared moment of serial consciousness.

Consciousness, it turns out, is what keeps us from being able to avoid an unwanted thought. The fact that our little window of consciousness can grasp, at once, both a thought and the metathought that wishes the thought away, means that it is forever caught in a paradox. We cannot split the thought from the metathought, even though this is the very purpose of the metathought. If the metathought is present, the thought is present; if the thought is absent, the metathought is absent. Consciousness embraces both the thought and the metathought at once—it allows us to think of them both. This means that in the long run, we can hope to suppress only *future* occurrences of a thought. Current consciousness is unable to think itself out of having a thought, because this entails thinking the thought. So, at best, our strategies must run toward the future in hopes that eventually the memory of what we set out to do will no longer dominate our thinking. We must think of what we should think about next, and try to arrange that this will not be the thought we are thinking now.

Successful suppression depends on our capacity to lose track of the metathought as well as the thought. Ironically, we must forget what we were doing, at least for a bit, if we wish to implement what we were doing. As a rule, we do this by changing to a new metathought—one directed toward thinking about something else. This is the strategy of *self-distraction,* and it is this strategy that is the concern of the next chapter. Because we cannot wish a thought away on the spot, we must look toward other things to capture our attention and draw our minds away.

FOUR

Self-Distraction

*"Oh, don't go on like that!" cried the poor Queen, wringing
her hands in despair. "Consider what a great girl you are.
Consider what a long way you've come today. Consider what
o'clock it is. Consider anything, only don't cry!"
Alice could not help laughing at this, even in the midst of her
tears. "Can you keep from crying by considering things?"
she asked.
"That's the way it's done," the Queen said with great decision:
"nobody can do two things at once, you know."*

—Lewis Carroll, *Through the Looking-Glass*

Distracting oneself seems easy enough. In fact, this is what
I've been doing all day prior to writing this chapter. First I
dawdled over coffee, read the newspaper, and became involved
in an unusually thorough tooth-flossing project. I used my own
teeth, so this didn't cause nearly the uproar or delay that it could
have. Then, I went to the office, read my mail, made a phone
call, and . . . hard to believe but it's three in the afternoon and
I have to quit soon to get the baby from the sitter's.
Procrastination is a kind of self-distraction, an engagement in
trivial activities when we wish to avoid a more important task
that looks too much like work.

Now that I've gotten myself started, I can point out that the
kind of self-distraction I did this morning was the easy kind. I
slipped into it without any planning or effort. When we wish
to avoid a disturbing unwanted thought, however, self-
distraction is not something we can do so naturally or effectively,

and it can escalate into a major chore. Try distracting yourself, for instance, when you are looking down from a great height, or when the itch of an insect bite is begging for a nice rough scratching. Self-distraction is one of the key strategies we use to keep our mind away from our fears, worries, secrets, forbidden ideas, and even itches, and for this reason it is important that we understand how to do it well.

Children are not very skilled at self-distraction, so they become quick victims to whatever grabs their attention. They can cry interminably as the result of a broken dolly, or become overwrought with a "boo boo" on their finger. They seem to be able to whine for hours about one thing, and always tend to become interested in what will soon spill or explode. Parents must learn, then, to supply distracters on a regular basis, helping the child to redirect attention away from things that can cause grief and toward more benign points of interest. After flying cross-country in a crowded plane with my toddler on my lap, I was convinced that the ability to distract is one of the great skills of parenting. All the passengers nearby agreed. The most effective parents I know are able to guide their children from the brink of hell to a state of bemused puttering in a matter of moments. Eventually, of course, the child must learn to do this for himself or herself, and self-distraction becomes one of the key abilities we have that gets us through adulthood—and through flights crowded with other people's children.

First we must understand the difference between direct suppression and self-distraction—two ways of trying to avoid an unwanted thought. We usually start with suppression, and then change our strategy to self-distraction. This step is a most important one, a transition we must make if we wish to suppress at all, and the chapter begins here. The next key issue is whether and when self-distraction can be expected to work. It may help sometimes and not others. So, we'll need to look at the different kinds of self-distraction, and whether they differ in their effectiveness in the fight against unwanted thoughts. Finally, we will consider the possibility that people build entire life-styles as a way of distracting themselves. Maybe people become totally absorbed in some things and oddly oblivious to others simply in the pursuit of peace of mind.

A Change of Plans. We have learned that "naked" suppression is not possible. Our mental apparatus is not built to clear itself, to think "I will not think of X" and then in fact immediately stop thinking of X forever. Indeed, it seems that the more energy we invest in the attempt to suppress, the more likely is the attempt to fail, landing us directly in that untidy spot in the road we were trying to step over. If all we ever did on encountering an unwanted thought, then, was to try direct suppression, we would make no progress at all. Trying not to think of X makes us think of X, as vividly, frequently, and efficiently as if we had decided to think of X from the start.

Suppression thus requires a mental transformation of the task. We move from "I will not think of X" to "I will think of Y." This is the basic form of self-distraction. It is a metacognitive strategy, a move from one way of metathinking about a thought to another. Admittedly, this mental transformation is a precarious one, in that trying to think of Y can remind us of why we undertook this task, and so bring us back to "avoid X."[54] However, the movement to "think of Y" has a number of benefits that can make it a useful first step in shaking loose the unwanted thought of X. In particular, the self-distractive thought does not automatically bring us back to X. Back when we were thinking "avoid X," the more effort we expended on our thought, the more it all backfired. But now in the "think Y" mode, the more cognitive effort we expend, the more we will focus on Y—and thus actually stay away from X.

This is a critical feature of self-distraction. As long as we attempt suppression only, then the harder we try, the deeper we get ourselves into the soup. When we attempt self-distraction, in contrast, our efforts can get us somewhere. Although we may still be reminded of the unwanted thought from time to time, there is at least some room in self-distraction for a brief respite, a time during which we can focus on something other than the unwanted idea. At least now, when we try harder to think, we do not find our thoughts defeating their own purposes. And it is in this time that our automatic perception and memory processes may edge the conscious window away from the whole mess, toward a more pleasing view that can hold our attention.

This way of understanding self-distraction helps us get a grip on the effects of stress and activity on unwanted thoughts. It helps us to understand why being busy (because of stress or just plain activity) can sometimes increase the occurrence of unwanted thoughts and at other times will seem to push them away. I've wondered about this a lot because of the odd things that vacations can do to my mental state. Sometimes going away and relaxing clears my mind wonderfully, whereas other times leaving the activities and stresses of my usual routine produces a unique sensitivity to worry and makes me wish I were home. The difference between these effects seems to hinge on whether one is trying to suppress or trying to self-distract.

Consider what happens when you go on vacation right after you have a major argument with your boss. With this nasty incident fresh in your mind, you set off to the beach. An argument like this has not happened before, so you probably have not had the occasion to try to distract yourself from such problems. In all likelihood, then, you will simply try to suppress the thought when you're on the vacation. And if so, you will find that you are refreshingly distracted by the water, the beach, and the surroundings. These things keep you from even trying to suppress the thought, and as a result the thought is swept away and you are left in peace. You wonder at this time how a vacation could ever *promote* an unwanted thought, and you scoff at the idea.

The next year, though, you go to the mountains. This time, the boss has been after you for some time to straighten up your act, and things at work are very unpleasant. To deal with this, you have taken to watching TV a lot at home and following the programs very carefully. Sure, it is not very exciting—but it keeps your mind off the mess at work and also keeps you up to date on all the fine bargains that your local retailers have to offer. In the cabin in the mountains, there is also a TV. But you don't watch it very much and instead you hike, take pictures, and enjoy the breathtaking views. Amidst all this, you find that the turmoil at work keeps coming to mind. You see a DON'T FEED THE BEARS sign and imagine your boss mauling a tourist. The vacation, rather than taking your mind off your worries, has taken your mind off your distractions—and so leaves you oddly worried even though you have come to "relax."

An important mental transition occurs when we change strategies—from the strategy of suppressing a thought to the strategy of distracting ourselves from that thought. This changes the rules by which external distractions influence the occurrence of unwanted thoughts. Such a rule change must be common, however, because when people are asked what they do to avoid unwanted thoughts, they mention self-distraction nearly every time.[55] And when people who identify themselves as chronic worriers are asked what they're doing wrong, they blame their inability to distract themselves from the targets of their worry.[56] The change from suppression to self-distraction is natural, the path we follow away from the thoughts we desire to avoid, but it also changes the way our mental efforts influence our thoughts. When we are suppressing, attention to what we are doing is injurious to our plan; when we are self-distracting, attention to what we are doing is exactly what we need.

Can Distraction Work?   Most of what we currently know about the effectiveness of distraction comes from experiments on pain. Dentists and physicians would love it if their patients would just stop whining, not to mention that the patients might be pleased as well, so pain control is an issue that has received a fair amount of scientific attention. In these studies, people are exposed to something painful—a real dental or surgical procedure, or a somewhat analogous discomfort such as keeping a hand in ice water for several minutes. They are asked to report when they begin to feel pain, how strong it is, whether they can continue, or the like, and these judgments are taken as measures of the degree of pain they are feeling. This is really all we have to go on, as there is no special "pain behavior" in the body that we can monitor to see how much discomfort the person is feeling. Wiggling and hopping and saying "Yipes!" are signs, but even they are unreliable at times.

If there is a general rule that emerges from pain studies, it is that distracters work best when they are absorbing.[57] For instance, music piped in during a dental procedure doesn't seem to make that much difference, whereas allowing the patient to play a video game reduces pain reports quite a bit.[58] You might argue that the kind of Muzak most dentists play can cause minor pain before you even sit in the chair. And it is true that a rendition of one's favorite music on a good stereo system might turn out to be more engaging than even a video game. These seemingly minor variations in the quality of the distracter could have a critical influence on the degree to which the distraction can hold one's attention away from the unwanted thought.

We should not make the mistake of assuming in all this that the distracter always needs to be pleasant. In one study, students who were asked to imagine having an argument with a callous professor showed more tolerance to ice water than those who did not distract themselves in this way.[59] At the extreme, there might even be some truth to the old joke about distracting oneself from a headache by stubbing one's toe. As one novelist observed, "a little pain cleans out the mind."[60] This even appears true when one pain clears our mind of another. In all likelihood, though, unpleasant distracters might not work if they were truly vile. In this case, we might begin trying to distract ourselves from *them,* and so lose whatever relief they were bringing.

Distracters can also be too challenging to work. Imagine trying to distract yourself from an insistent backache, for example, by reviewing Einstein's work for errors. The distracter is too difficult to allow total absorption, and the pain overtakes the mind. This problem with self-distraction was shown in one study when people were asked to perform one of several different arithmetic tasks while their hands were immersed in ice water.[61] Those who simply repeated a series of digits felt the pain, whereas those who were asked to add digits in their heads and verbalize the result reported less pain sensation. Yet another group was asked to add digits and then classify the result as above 50 and odd or below 50 and even, or as another number. This group felt the pain, too, probably because the task was so difficult they couldn't become fully engaged in it. Quite simply, it appears we need distracters that are neither too difficult nor too easy; we prefer ones that just match what we can do.

Distraction is not, however, the perfect solution for all pain. You have probably experienced certain pains in your life that you swear you could not be distracted from even if the Rolling Stones played a concert in your sinuses. Pain can be too great, too insistent and annoying, to allow any relief through distraction. With this in mind, it makes sense to learn that, on occasion, people report less pain when they actually *focus attention* on the painful sensation than when they attempt distraction. Women who were asked to monitor their internal sensations during labor, for example, in one study reported less pain than women asked to distract themselves.[62] This strategy may be better for severe pain, even though distraction is more effective for mild pain.[63]

Severe pains appear to "break through" the shield of self-distraction, no matter how absorbed we have become with our distracting thoughts. It may be that attending to the pain works best in these cases because it saves us the added anguish that occurs when we continually try to distract ourselves and fail. Repeated botched attempts to think of other things can only make us resentful, discouraged, and irritable. In cases of severe pain, then, the best thing to do may be to give up self-distraction, go ahead and think about the pain, and perhaps in this way eliminate the turmoil in our mind that accompanies the painful feelings.

If it is true that pain is a good analog of all our unwanted thoughts, then we can draw some lessons from this research. In general, for instance, it seems that we should be very careful in selecting our distracters when we have unwanted thoughts. We should find distracters that will last, that can engage us and draw our attention for a long time without leaving us confused or bored. And we may not be able to trust self-distraction when our unwanted thoughts are extremely urgent and insistent. Like severe pain, severely disturbing thoughts may drag us back to face them each time we wish them away. Self-distraction is likely to be an ineffective strategy, adding only more distress to the mental mixture because of its repeated failure.

Focused and Unfocused Self-Distraction. Most psychological studies of distraction call for people to think about a single distracter. People are asked to imagine a pleasant scene, listen to music, or the like. Such instructions do not reflect very well what people actually do, however, when they attempt to distract themselves from unwanted thoughts. In the throes of the mental turmoil that accompanies an unwanted thought, most people seem unable to keep coming back to one distracter. Rather, they report that their minds "race" and "spin," and they appear to touch on multiple distracters in turn. Whenever one distracter fails for an instant, and the unwanted thought surfaces, the person typically *changes* to a new distracter.

This suggests that most studies of distraction are irrelevant to the real strategies people use. Traditional studies have examined only *focused* self-distraction, the attempt to think of one item or a relatively circumscribed topic. What people really do when they fight unwanted thoughts is instead to call in all the troops; they seek one distracter after another in the forlorn hope that something will finally grab their attention and wrest it away from the thought they abhor. *Unfocused* self-distraction seems to be the rule rather than the exception. To avoid an unwanted thought, the person skips rapidly from one distracter to another, seldom repeating. The individual does what a character in Dostoevsky's *Crime and Punishment* did just prior to committing suicide: "Avidly he looked to the right and to the left, staring intently at every object, yet finding nothing on which he could fasten his attention."

People trying not to think of a white bear show a similar lack of focus. The typical participant in a thought suppression study of this kind, you will recall, is asked to think aloud while attempting to suppress the thought of a white bear. The person may spend a bit of time trying not to think, experimenting with simple suppression, but then usually moves to a self-distraction strategy. The person may say, "I'll think about this desk," for example, and then carry on describing the desk or recalling memories that are suggested by this topic. Soon, however, the person tires of desk talk, and the white bear returns. At this time, the person then says, "Okay, I'll think about my favorite shoehorns," or some such, and sets off again on a brief monologue on this topic. When the white bear returns later on, the person usually jumps to yet a new distracter in the next attempt to suppress.

The tactic of unfocused self-distraction seems natural enough. Why should someone return to focus on an old distracter that evidently didn't work last time? The trouble is, changing focus over and over may be responsible for later preoccupation with the suppression topic. Recall that in the white bear studies, people who are invited to think about a white bear after a period of suppressing it usually become especially obsessed. They mention it more than do people who are merely asked to think about it from the start. It may be that unfocused self-distraction during suppression sets in motion a chain of events that produces this rebound effect.

Unfocused self-distraction, after all, is a particularly fine way of thinking about many different things. Each item one brings to mind as a distracter is considered briefly, then the unwanted thought pops in, and the distracter is rejected. This happens repeatedly, and the result is that many different things perceived in one's immediate environment, and memories that are easily retrieved, become known as *not white bears*. These things are nonetheless thought about in rapid alternation with thoughts of a white bear. And the wide-ranging review of one's current thoughts for something to distract oneself from a white bear makes all these thoughts likely later to be reminders of a white bear. When one stops suppressing and turns instead to thinking about the white bear, this thinking is made unusually easy by the many cues to the topic that are available in the room and in recent memory. The physical surroundings, and many other things that come to mind, are vaguely reminiscent of the thought that was earlier unwanted, so the thought is prompted again and again.

Red Volkswagen. An experiment was conducted to see whether focused self-distraction can in fact eliminate the rebound of an unwanted thought.[64] The people in this study were presented with the same situation as those in the original white bear experiment, with one exception. Some participants who were asked to try not to think of a white bear were also instructed to use a single distracter whenever a white bear happened to come to mind. They were asked to focus on a red Volkswagen instead. This instruction was planned to subvert people's more usual tendency to float from one distracter to another, and it did so quite successfully. Those participants given this instruction mentioned red Volkswagen several times during the suppression period—usually just after mentioning white bear.

Using a focused distracter didn't help people much during suppression. The red Volkswagen group indicated thinking about the unwanted white bear about as much as another group of participants who were allowed to use the natural, unfocused self-distraction tactic. But the red VW group escaped the re-

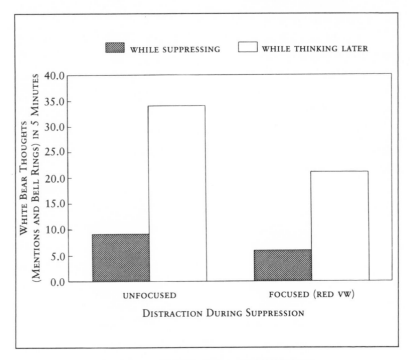

Figure 1. WHITE BEAR THOUGHTS

bound effect. The tendency to talk profusely about white bears after suppression, observed as usual in the participants who used their own unfocused strategy, was not at all evident in the red VW group (see Figure 1). Those participants who had focused on a single distracter showed no special tendency to become preoccupied with the original unwanted thought, the white bear.

These findings have important implications for the success of self-distraction. It appears that focusing on a single distracter produces little immediate relief; it wasn't any easier for subjects in this study to avoid thinking about a white bear if they consistently focused on a red VW. But the longer-term advantages of this strategy were clear. Thinking about a single item, even a random one like a red VW, seems to prevent the normal consequence of self-distraction, the mental linking of the unwanted thought to every distracting idea that comes by. So, when one is allowed to think of the unwanted thought, the immediate mental territory is not a set of thoughts recently linked to white bear. Rather, one's conscious thoughts are relatively uncontaminated by association with the unwanted thought.

The red VW, of course, *is* contaminated. The focused distracter is likely to be a very strong reminder of the unwanted thought. Fortunately, however, you can put a distracter like this one away. Unless there is a red VW in the room, or one tattooed on your arm, there is likely to be little reason to dwell on that reminder and so return to the white bear. The red VW, in a sense, serves as a "lightning rod" that absorbs the recurrent unwanted white bear thoughts and keeps them from striking everything else on your mind. So, rather than a torched mental landscape, you are left with only a lightning-struck red VW. When it is kept in the garage, there is later no damage to be seen.

There are some everyday parallels to this artificially induced strategy. Items that children seek for "security," for example—such as blankets or stuffed animals (even white bears)—could have the same palliative influence we found with the red VW. Returning to a familiar comfort whenever you encounter an undesirable thought may reduce your tendency to seek many different distracters. Some people report, for example, that whenever they have an unwanted thought, they pray or think of God. This is a focused self-distraction strategy that, like turning to thoughts of a red VW, may produce long-term advances in the avoidance of the unwanted thought.

There is the possibility, though, that the focused distracter could over time itself become a strong reminder of many unwanted thoughts. Then, you may need special convincing to approach the distracter itself. Perhaps people who pray only when they're in trouble come eventually to dislike their God. If you are going to pray, turn to a familiar object or idea, or otherwise seek a single focus for self-distraction, it might be desirable on occasion to "cleanse" that focus by thinking about it in good times or in a positive light. Perhaps this is one of the things church services are for. The good feelings a person gets at church might be helpful in removing the tarnish of unwanted thoughts from the religious ideas the person has used as distracters.

As a final note on red Volkswagens, we should point out that these observations help us find some redeeming value in psychological research on distraction. Although we were complaining just a bit ago about the tendency of researchers to ignore the most common strategy people use on themselves—unfocused distraction—it now turns out researchers did investigate the tactic that probably works the best—focused distraction. They may not have known this when they started out, but they happen to have hit on the right one.

The Pursuit of Absorption.   All the indications we have considered to this point in the chapter suggest one thing: If we wish to suppress a thought, it is necessary to become absorbed in another thought. The distracter we seek should be something intrinsically interesting and engaging to us, and even if it is unpleasant, should not be boring or confusing. This is not a good description of a red Volkswagen. That distracter was chosen merely as an odd thought to bring focus to a person's self-distraction attempts in one study. A lasting, useful theme for self-distraction will probably need to be more extensive than that.

How can we become absorbed in something? One way to think about this is to examine what it is that interests people most. No, I'm not talking about sex, although that is certainly a candidate. The things that interest people most are the things that provide good exercise for their abilities. The things that do not interest us, in turn, are those that are beyond our abilities or are much below our abilities. This general idea has been expressed in a theory of the "flow" experience.[65] According to this theory, we are most absorbed, interested, and entertained when we are doing something that precisely matches our capabilities. When this happens, we experience a psychological state of flow, a total engagement with what we are doing.

The good tennis player who takes on someone of equal ability, for example, will usually become absorbed with the game. The child who has just learned to cut paper dolls, too, may well become engaged in the experience. Many people find this kind of engagement in their work—if it is a proper challenge for them. Even washing dishes can be absorbing and interesting if you find it to be a challenge that just matches your abilities. This theory indicates, then, that there is nothing intrinsically interesting about anything. Rather, the proper match between the person and the activity is what produces engagement.

When the person is too good at the task, boredom sets in. Most of us experience little flow when we wash dishes, for instance, even with all that running water, because we are so good at this there is little danger we will not succeed. And once the child has cut the six hundredth paper doll, the joy may no longer spring from this task. The child may complain of the continuing danger of paper cuts and attempt to quit work. The opposing possibility, of course, is that your ability will not be sufficient to perform the task. So, the very first time you try to make conversation with an attractive stranger, you may be quite far from flow, ready instead to evacuate the room at the first opportunity. When your abilities are not up to your activities, anxiety and tension take over and spoil it all.

The odd implication of this theory is that we will never be satisfied. Normally, people get better at things the more they do them. Thus, just as we are getting our abilities to the point of a flow experience with some activity, and so pass the early anxieties of failure, we find ourselves improving so much that we are now bored with the entire thing. To remain continually absorbed, we need to keep making our jobs harder, revising our ambitions to match our advancing skills. In essence, although we may be doing the same thing over and over, we need to raise our standards as we proceed, and so arrange over time to continue in flow.

This way of thinking about absorption may seem most suited to the case of the workaholic. It is easy to envision setting higher and higher goals at work, and so becoming absorbed with your occupation. But absorption is not only a property of careers. You can become absorbed in almost all the activities of daily life—with the proper goal-setting. Next time you are wrestling with an unwanted thought as you perform some humdrum daily task, you might consider revising that task to make it more absorbing. Instead of cooking the same recipe to the point that you can find the ingredients in your sleep, for instance, you might try a new recipe, or experiment with the old one. Revisions of tasks that are currently boring you might pave the way for absorption and effective self-distraction. At worst, you only risk poisoning your family.

The opposing strategy would be useful for tasks that are currently too difficult. If some activity usually causes you anxiety, and so thwarts any attempt to become absorbed in it, perhaps you need to make the task smaller or sharpen your skills in this area. You might be trying to "impress the boss," for example, and find this very difficult to do. If you revise it to be a bit less ambitious—say, only to "get the work done on time"—then it may become something that in fact matches your current abilities. There is good evidence from a number of experiments that cutting back the definition of a task can help people to perform better when they find the task difficult. The actual activity doesn't change, only the way it is identified.[66] Then, instead of being a dreaded interlude that gives rise to anxiousness and unwanted thoughts, the work becomes something you can do and in which you can become absorbed.

It feels good to be absorbed. We seek absorption even when we have not consciously formulated a plan to become absorbed and we engage in actions designed to keep us in that state and away from the boredom or anxiety that follow when we leave it. Perhaps the pursuit of absorption is a lifetime activity for us all. It is fun to be in flow, and this experience should generally shield us from all but the most insistent unwanted thoughts. In effect, when we are absorbed in what we are doing, we are immunized against unwanted thoughts. Following this idea to its conclusion, then, suggests that much of what we do could be motivated by the avoidance of unwanted thoughts. The reason we become immersed in our work, in our romantic exploits, in our friends, in our hobbies, in our children—in every absorbing aspect of life—could be that we are avoiding thinking about disturbing things.

Freud would certainly have appreciated this kind of analysis. He argued that many of our seemingly noble activities are only stopgaps, replacements for the satisfaction of sexual and aggressive impulses that we deny ourselves. And at the extreme, a life of self-distraction could be characterized in this way. It is with this somewhat unsavory notion in mind that we should take a step back and evaluate self-distraction once again. Certainly, self-distraction is helpful in many cases of mental anguish. We need it, and at times we need to do it as effectively as we can. But self-distraction is also a brand of self-deception, a way in which we can lie to ourselves. Can that be best for us in the long run?

The Pursuit of Oblivion. Self-distraction has the property of being a negative or subtractive motivation, a desire not to think, not to feel, not to do, not to be. Taken to its logical conclusion, self-distraction could leave us with no real "self" at all, nothing we can genuinely say we are or want to become. Everything we think becomes a substitute, a poor second. If the avoidance of thoughts and feelings were all that motivated us through life, we would consider our lives complete successes if we dried up and blew away. There would be nothing at all to look forward to, except perhaps the ability to get into smaller clothing sizes.

Self-distraction has the potential to make us oblivious, not just about particular thoughts, but about ourselves as a whole. When people learn something unpleasant about themselves, for instance, they may not only avoid thinking about the unpleasant fact, they may come for a time to avoid thinking about themselves entirely. People in one experiment who had just failed a test, for instance, spent less time than others afterwards looking at themselves in a mirror.[67] Men in another study who had just been rejected by an attractive woman became unwilling to listen to their own tape-recorded voice.[68] Anything that reminds us of an unwanted thought, even our own image or voice, can be the target for self-distraction.

Unfortunately, such wholesale self-avoidance can have dire effects. We can become mean and heartless, not just toward others[69] but toward ourselves as well.[70] An unwillingness to think about ourselves would seem to be the first step toward rejoining the less enlightened members of the animal kingdom. It is our ability to reflect on ourselves, to gauge what we are, and to aspire to what we wish to be, that distinguishes us as self-conscious and morally responsible creatures. Anything that threatens to block permanently this ability to attend to ourselves imperils this most desirable and essential human characteristic. The urge to distract ourselves from an unwanted thought can serve to start just such a rush toward oblivion.

It is thus possible to blame many human ills on self-distraction run wild. When the attempt to distract oneself becomes no longer a conscious strategy, but instead an automatic and recurrent response to a problem, it can become more of a problem than the problem. People who have become dangerously zealous about a bizarre idea, for instance, may be pursuing absorption in this area to find oblivion somewhere else. It is hard not to suspect that when someone becomes extraordinarily interested in something boring, deeply involved in something shallow, or highly positive toward something negative, there may be an attempt at self-distraction pressing from the rear. Actions that are carried on without visible means of support can blind us to ourselves, leaving us without the ability to correct our patterns of action and thought.

A horrifying example of such self-estrangement can be found in Adolf Eichmann, the Nazi officer convicted in 1961 of "crimes against humanity" for his role in the Holocaust. The story of his trial told by Hannah Arendt is called *Eichmann in Jerusalem: A Report on the Banality of Evil*,[71] and it aptly reveals a shallow, distracted man. He entered the military having little idea of what the Nazis were up to, and spent his time working out the details of transportation, deportation, and eventually, extermination of the Jews. He was a bureaucrat, obsessed with orders and duties and making sure his actions were exactly what his superiors wanted, no less and no more. He spoke in clichés and repeated himself often. He showed little if any recognition of the magnitude of his atrocities, and claimed that disobedience to Hitler was more "unthinkable" than any of his actions against the Jews. The judges at his trial told him all he had said was "empty talk"—except that they thought the emptiness was false, and that he was hoping to cover up other thoughts that were far less empty, but more hideous.

Amidst this, there were signs of his inner turmoil. Most striking is his statement "I will jump into my grave laughing, because the fact that I have the death of five million Jews on my conscience gives me extraordinary satisfaction."[72] This statement, at once a wild, erroneous boast and a claim extremely out of character for such an unenthusiastic man, was something he began to say to his men near the end of the war—and then kept repeating *ad nauseam* to anyone who would listen, even years later in Argentina and again at his trial. It is as though once he could no longer distract himself from the enormity of his deeds, he could only proclaim them insanely. Most of our unwanted thoughts pale in comparison to what this man held back, but the lesson we can learn is the same. Self-distraction practiced for more than a short while can cloud our minds and deprive us of our judgment.

Self-distraction is best as a quick reaction, the first aid in a psychological emergency. But Band-Aids and aspirin and hot soup won't do forever. In some cases, they may even impede the healing or self-correction processes that should go on. The broadest message of the chapter is this: Although self-distraction can be used to escape unwanted thoughts in the short run, it is probably not the strategy of choice for reaching a satisfying and effective solution to the problem that created the unwanted thoughts in the first place. Reaching that solution will require, at least as a first step, a return to thinking about the unwanted thought. Such confrontation is rarely *all* that is needed, however, since just thinking the thought over and over is likely to produce nothing but distress.

Facing the unwanted thought, however, is a beginning. You must know your enemy to fight it, and self-distraction amounts to little more than running away. Research on people who have made some form of self-distraction into a habit indicates that self-distraction is indeed only a quick fix. People who generally avoid thinking about stresses seem to get along better than others right after the stressor hits, but those who by nature attend to the stress fare better later on.[73] So, self-distraction works at first, and it is better than paying attention to the unwanted thought. But eventually, it becomes important to return your attention to the problem and find a solution. Putting the thought out of mind is not the same as putting the problem it represents out of existence.

FIVE

The Remote Control of Thinking

A grateful environment is a substitute for happiness. It can quicken us from without just as a fixed hope and affection, or the consciousness of a right life, can quicken us from within.

—George Santayana, *The Sense of Beauty*

Have you ever treated yourself as if you were someone else? Playing a game of chess or backgammon against yourself would be a clear example, but most people don't do this very often. More commonplace instances include writing notes to yourself, laying out clothes for yourself the night before a hurried morning, or placing a photo of a fat person on the refrigerator in hopes of scaring yourself away. In each of these cases, you assume that your current state of mind is different enough from the one you will be in later for you to treat the subsequent "you" almost like a different person. You arrange circumstances now that will have an impact on you later. When that time comes, you may look back and think, Gosh, how thoughtful of me, or, That old gambit? How stupid do I think I *am,* anyway?

Sometimes these little tricks we play on ourselves seem downright silly. At other times, however, they can be very helpful and effective. Their common quality is that they require an abandonment of the usual *internal* control we exercise over our thoughts, emotions, and actions, and a reorientation toward the *external* control of these things. But we do not leave this external control up to chance. We take control of ourselves by arranging external events so that later we will have to behave in accord with them. This, then, is a kind of remote control, a way of operating ourselves—choosing our directions for thought—by choosing the circumstances we will subsequently encounter and trusting that these circumstances will influence us.

This chapter is about this circuitous form of mental control. We will begin by exploring why anyone would ever want to do this. Then we will look into how remote control works, what exactly it is we can do to make our circumstances control our thoughts so we can relax. People seem to use this technique both in attempts to concentrate on things and in attempts to suppress things, and the technique can lead either to mental stability or to change. But there are some catches in this kind of self-control that can hinder our progress, subtle obstacles that get in our way when we ignore the powerful effects that our circumstances—both chosen and unchosen—can have on our thinking.

The Costs of Control. Keeping direct, internal control over our thoughts can sometimes amount to a terrible chore. Like the juggler spinning plates at the circus, we find ourselves in great difficulty trying to keep all the plates going at once, and we start to break a few. Maybe more than a few. Trying to keep our mind in order as we must simultaneously deal with many other thought processes that require conscious attention means that sometimes we fail to control our behaviors—we leave our coat in the cab, shake salt in our coffee, or forget a key appointment. We cannot watch everything at once, and this is the reason we resort to playing elaborate tricks on ourselves.

Controlling everything is not always a problem, because, as we have learned, certain mental tasks take place automatically and thus do not interfere with one another. We can relax and leave breathing up to the automatic pilot, for instance, secure in knowing we will not forget to breathe if we ignore direct control.[74] But if we are trying to do something that does require considerable conscious attention, and we are not yet so practiced at it that it can carry on automatically, it may fail in the face of simultaneous demands on our attention from elsewhere. There are many cases of this kind of conflict, but some particularly intriguing ones have recently been discovered by social psychologists.

Imagine, for instance, that you are trying to lie to someone. (For a worthy cause, of course.) Normally, a lie requires some thought suppression. You must not think too much about the truth, for instance, or that will get in the way. You should not think too much about the fact that it is a lie, either, because this might find its way into your conversation, too. And there is your body to think about as well. Suppress any incorrect facial expressions, postures, or gestures; don't give yourself away by snickering or putting your hand over your eyes and peeking out through your fingers. The act of lying, in short, may require a notable amount of attention directed toward suppression.

Add to this mix, now, an unusually strong motive to make the lie work. Say, for instance, your job is on the line and you must convince the boss that you were not responsible for the food fight in the cafeteria yesterday. This extra motivation adds even more to think about. Now, you must consider what will happen if the boss sees through the ruse—how everyone will look at you as you skulk away with your belongings, what it will be like to apply for work elsewhere with this on your record. Visions of yourself homeless, warming your hands at a barrel fire, clog your mind just as you are trying to place the key embellishments on your lie.

Then something happens: You squirm, or use the wrong tone of voice, or pause too long, or perhaps not long enough—and you know it is over. The boss sees through it all, and you are out of work. Research on deception indicates that too much motivation to deceive can have exactly this ironic effect.[75] With too many reasons to lie, people "leak" the truth more often, defeating their own attempts to deceive by giving nonverbal signs that they are lying. This, then, is a clear case when the attempt at direct, internal control of oneself can cause an overload of conscious attention, and subsequent failure to control key behaviors and their effects. It is a good example of the general rule that when we are busy or bothered, we have difficulty keeping up a false front for the benefit of others.[76]

Another undesirable consequence of direct attempts at suppression is that they can lead us to make superficial judgments of other people. Normally, it can take some careful thought about other people to reach valid conclusions about why they do what they do. When such thought is interrupted by a conscious attempt to suppress something, it is easy to reach incorrect conclusions about others. Suppose, for instance, you are being questioned by the police about something you did. There are two officers in the room, and one begins by being blunt and abusive. You steel yourself through this and say nothing incriminating. However, he then stands very close to you with his fists clenched while the second one asks some questions in a kind, normal tone. Although these guys are obviously using the "good cop, bad cop" ploy to try to get you to crack, a time-worn strategy that is often prompted by just this situation, you are taken in completely. You decide that the second fellow really is on your side and you spill the beans to him.

They kept you busy suppressing worries about the "bad cop" and so led you to make an incorrect inference about the "good cop"—and thus to confess. An experiment was conducted on such processes, and it showed that suppression can indeed promote faulty interpersonal judgments. The study called for people to try to discern why a man they had just met was answering political questions in a strongly conservative manner.[77] If you saw someone making conservative statements and you had no other information, you would probably guess that he was conservative. But the participants in this experiment were given some very important information: It was revealed to them that this man had been given a set of conservative answers to read by the experimenters. So anyone judging his personal degree of liberal versus conservative leanings should say: "Reading prepared conservative statements as a favor to the experimenters is no indication of his political leanings, so I'd say the best guess is that he is moderate."

To arrange for some participants to suppress and others not to suppress, a clever circumstance was devised. Participants were initially introduced to this individual under special conditions: For some, he acted pleasant and polite, making a good impression, whereas for others this same gentleman acted abrasive and aloof, and so made a decidedly bad impression. Then some participants were asked to try to ingratiate themselves with him while others were asked only to watch. Now, attempting to be nice to someone whom you do not like is perhaps the epitome of social circumstances that occasion thought suppression. One is smiling on the surface, making nice-nice, and holding back the desire for a rolled-up newspaper to give the jerk a good swat.

The people who were encouraged to suppress in this way needed to spend much of their conscious attention controlling their thoughts about the interaction. As a result, they drew the completely inappropriate inference from the gentleman's answers to the political questions. They decided he was conservative—even though everyone was told from the start that he hadn't even made up the answers himself and was simply asked to read them. The suppressing subjects, in trying to be nice to a nasty man, arrived at the most shallow inferences about his personality. Perhaps if he had been standing on one leg, they would have mistaken him for a flamingo.

The lesson of such research is that internal control is costly.

It can consume important cognitive capacity and leave us behaving foolishly because so little of our conscious mind can be devoted to the other tasks that confront us. Although it is probably inevitable that we will get into scrapes like these from time to time, there is no need to make this a continuous battle. Occasionally, we can transfer internal control to external sources, and so leave ourselves with more mental room for everyday tactical thinking. If we could just avoid the boss, for instance, or observe the "conservative" man from a distance, we could sidestep the confusion that occurs when we try to control too much at once. We can stop working to concentrate or suppress—to bring our mind nearer some things and farther away from others. One way to do this is to approach or avoid—and so bring our body nearer some things and farther away from others.

People, Places, and Things. The items in our lives that prompt thoughts can be generally classified as "cues" for thinking. The people we know, the places we go, and the objects we find all act as cues and call to mind various thoughts. To gain remote control over our thinking, then, requires that we gain some control over these cues for our thought. If we can make them closer when we want to be reminded by them, or farther away when we wish to suppress the thoughts they can prompt, then we have achieved the remote control of our minds.[78] This kind of control can be much more lasting, powerful, and indeed, irrevocable than the internal variety.

When I want to think about something, say a scientific problem, I try to get near something that will continually remind me of it. This might be a book on a relevant topic, for example, or it might be a person to whom I want to talk about it, or merely a section of the library to go sit in. I may not even read the book very carefully, as I drift off to think of the problem I want to solve; later, when I look at my jottings in the margins, they may have little to do with the book at all. And unfortunately, I may also fail to pay attention to a person I'm with, as I've become caught up in my own thoughts about the problem we're "discussing" and have not really listened. The spot in the library could also be ignored, serving only to help me keep my mind off other things that would be prompted by the exciting jumble of cues available elsewhere.

The use of cues for concentration is a common and easily used strategy for everyone, not just absentminded professors like me. An interesting example is the photographs people use to help remind them of special things they wish to be able to think about again. We commonly take more pictures at weddings and celebrations than at other times, and take more pictures of babies and children than of adults.[79] Apparently, when we are going through periods of great change, we try to capture moments along the way for later thought. These photos then seem to take on a life of their own as reminders of the way we were. One can even begin to reconstruct the past around the photos, leaving out events or people that are not pictured and overemphasizing those that are, merely because the external cues are so powerful.

People also use the control of thinking cues to induce suppression. Right after breaking up with a lover or a spouse, for example, it is not unheard of for people to avoid their old haunts. You might avoid the place where the partner lived, for instance, or places where you went together. Photos might be discarded, objects you bought together might find their way to the Goodwill store, and friends you shared might even be shed in the attempt to avoid reminders. All this might leave you feeling even more lonely than before, stripped of many of the old, familiar things in your life, but it could be worth it nonetheless for the mental peace that comes as a result.

Years later, however, you might look back and notice that you have a missing chapter in that part of your life history. Although Freud and others might want to argue that you had been the victim of repression, the unconsciously motivated forgetting of threatening material, this would not adequately describe what had happened. Rather than a simple "going blank," and erasure of items from memory, this apparent repression is traceable instead to an active avoidance. The avoidance of people, places, and things associated with an unwanted thought, over time, reduces dramatically the number of times you are required by your circumstance to deal with relevant information, and this promotes forgetting.

In the case of the old flame, for example, your avoidance of common friends, places, and shared objects eliminates many instances in which you must retrieve the flame's name or characteristics from memory. Talking about the former partner is reduced to a minimum, so generating information about the partner and learning new things about him or her is made infrequent as well. There is thus an absence of the usual "refreshing" of memory that we experience in the case of people and events we think and talk about a lot. The flame grows cold not because we've doused it but because we have failed to fuel the fire. We experience memory loss, then, not by virtue of an internal thought process, but in consequence of the long-term effects of a remote control process.[80]

This is a behavioral repression, then, rather than a mental one. We forget by avoiding people, places, or things in the world, whenever we have trouble avoiding these reminders in our minds. In all likelihood, real forgetting does occur in these circumstances, but it occurs in the same way you forget the names of your high school classmates or the lineup of the Tigers in '77. Unless you review the high school yearbook on a regular basis, or fondly recite the Tigers' batting averages for fun each day, these items fade from memory. They are not actively used. The tactic we use to introduce external control of unwanted thoughts, then, takes advantage of the fact that our minds require exercise in an area to maintain live connections to that area. When we avoid cues behaviorally, we come to avoid thoughts almost as well as if we had shut off the thoughts themselves.

Of course, there are some problems with this. One young man who had a particularly difficult time breaking up with a woman confided to me that he was saddened for a time by all other women. They didn't serve as distracters, but rather as reminders. Each time he would see someone else, he would find some inflection in her voice, some feature of her past, that would remind him of the love he lost. For a while, then, he ended up avoiding all women in the pursuit of remote control over his grief. Taken to the extreme, his strategy could prove remarkably confining. In the attempt to achieve control over a thought, one might seclude oneself from *most* cues—people, places, and things—and live the life of a hermit. This strategy might then backfire, as a life isolated from everything would seem to be a breeding ground for every unwanted thought one could imagine.

The further difficulty with resorting to external control is that its effects can be hard to reverse. Unlike our minds, our worlds once changed can be impossible to change back. When we avoid people who remind us of a painful thought, they may read our absence as animosity toward them, and so make it very difficult to resume the relationship. Or, when we choose a particular life setting as a control strategy—say, joining the foreign legion to forget a spoiled romance—we may well be stuck with the new situation for much longer than we had expected. Throwing away objects that remind us of unwanted thoughts can also be far too precipitous a response, especially when we learn that the objects were valuable. The great charm of remote control is that it can be irreversible in this way, helping us to control our minds in a way that we never could from within. But this is its great danger as well. We often shrink from remote control, choosing continued mental control in circumstances that keep echoing unwanted thoughts, because changing the external world can be so final.

Using Order and Disorder.   Our emphasis so far has been on two relatively straightforward directions for external control—approach and avoidance. We have noted primarily that approaching cues that remind us of something can yield concentration, whereas avoidance of such cues can produce suppression. These techniques work because at the most elementary level, our minds often operate as direct reflections of what impinges on our senses. What's coming in through our senses is directly projected on our conscious experience, and so influences our thoughts. There may be more subtle processes underlying such effects, however, systems of remote control that depend for their operation on more than the simple presence or absence of external stimuli.

Consider the case of your closet. Like me, you probably have some very favorite clothes that hang in the most accessible area. You wear these more than the others, and when it comes time to put on something else, you may even have to search a bit to find what you want. Still, you may have an organized arrangement with sections for pants, shirts or blouses, and so on, so the search ends fairly soon. I notice that the old stuff I never wear, and never again expect to wear, is not organized in these sections. Rather, it is in the back in disarray. If I wanted to find one thing in that area, I would have to haul out everything.

Could it be we manage to suppress sometimes by leaving certain cues disorganized in our lives? Like the items in the back of the closet, the reminders of an unwanted thought are left in physical disarray, and so cannot serve as strong external goads to renew our thinking. I tend to do this with old research projects that have gone awry. Instead of gathering all the data and computer analyses together and labeling them properly so I can find them again, I leave everything scattered. Some things are in the lab, others in a file drawer, and yet others I've entrusted to an assistant who happens to have moved to Milwaukee. Without really admitting it to myself, I've decided that the project is going nowhere. Then, I guarantee that by leaving it a mess.

The perception that your external cues are disorganized tends to reduce your confidence that the external information can be found.[81] It is not only for academics and others who must maintain access to lots of information that this is important. It pops up everywhere. The use of disorganization seems a strong candidate for "sneaky trick on yourself of the month," a broad scheme for the remote control of thinking. Unwanted thoughts of running out of money can be dispelled by keeping your checkbook in total disarray. Unwanted thoughts of a broken relationship can be avoided by allowing reminders to dissipate in every direction. Unwanted thoughts of a disease can be set aside for a time by losing your pills or misplacing the doctor's number.

You probably know people who seem to use this scheme to suppress, and you may have used it as well. Organization and disorganization have strong effects on our memory abilities, and it would not be surprising if we used this fact as a tactic for self-control. It is interesting to note, though, that the fully conscious and deliberate use of such a strategy may undermine its usefulness; if you were to mess up your closet deliberately, you would probably remember very clearly where each "disorganized" item had been placed. Organizing something consciously may aid in later concentration, but disorganizing to suppress probably works only when you "let it happen" rather than plan it out in detail. Indeed, it is unclear whether the use of organization and disorganization is commonly a conscious strategy at all. Sometimes we seem to do these things automatically, or even just as side effects of using or failing to use a body of information, and when this happens it is hard to maintain that a planned strategy is being employed.

There is at least one case, though, in which putting things in order is a highly strategic and planned path to mental control. I know I become a mad listmaker before any major trip; my wife is reassured by lists too, and once we even made a list of all the lists we made. The comfort that comes from these activities is in direct proportion to the degree to which internal mental control activities are replaced by external devices. Before going to Europe one summer, for example, I found I kept having thoughts that were partly wanted and partly unwanted. The thought of "remember the Chap Stick" would come to mind (as though there are no people with lips in all of Europe), and though I'd want to remember to pack it, I'd also not really need to be thinking this while driving down the freeway to work. So I'd put it off, hoping it would come back later. On finally making the list, of course, I was then haunted by the possibility that there were crucial items that I had put off writing down and had now forgotten. I can only report that the list, once "complete," saved me from much needless rehearsal and mental unrest.

Connection and Disconnection. Another subtle form of remote control is based on a different principle of memory. It is generally true that thinking about an item's relationship to other things—a process of *elaboration*—is likely to enhance memory for that item.[82] We tend to do this quite automatically as we encounter new ideas we wish to remember. We meet Aunt Theresa for the first time, for instance, and immediately we think how she resembles someone we know (in this case, Abraham Lincoln). Later on, the connections formed in this way may help us remember her—as we see her face on every penny we handle. It is natural to elaborate on incoming information, and as we do this we create ways to get back to it when we next need it.

To concentrate on a thought using elaboration as a remote control tactic, all you would need to do is forge mental links between the thought and whatever else is handy. Writing the name or initials of a school "crush" all over your notebooks, locker, and desk, for example, is likely to promote much subsequent thinking about the secret love. Any activity that brings the desired thought into juxtaposition with many other thoughts, especially those you are likely to encounter later on, will promote concentration. By the same token, an effort to stop elaboration is likely to be helpful as a suppression tactic. The way to prevent elaborative links from being formed between an unwanted thought and the many people, places, and things in your life is the *physical isolation* of those things that are already reminders.

This technique keeps us from making connections between our unwanted thought and the other thoughts we often have. For instance, you might attempt to suppress thoughts of a painful relationship with a relative by keeping all traces of him or her in one place. All the letters from Aunt Theresa, photos of her, and gifts from her are kept in a box in the closet. Although they are highly organized and accessible in an instant, they are also quarantined, kept apart from other belongings and mementos. In that way, you never connect them in your mind with the other segments of your life. The major portion of your surroundings can thus be thought about without danger of elaborative connections that bring your thinking back to the awful aunt. Just like disorganization, extreme organization—and sequestering—can serve as a remote control device to disconnect us from our unwanted thoughts.

These subtle techniques for the self-control of thinking may be important forces that shape our environments. We usually see the room, house, car, office, friends, family, and possessions that people have as reflections of their past, indications of what they have accumulated in life and how they have preserved their own history. An appreciation of the remote control of thinking suggests, in contrast, that these things may have been arranged primarily with a view toward the future. The individual's selection of persons, places, and things may be a slowly and subtly built structure for thinking, a structure that keeps in some thoughts and keeps out others. It is assembled on purpose to ensure future mental peace. All of this then saves the person the constant trouble of having to exert mental control in search of a particular desired pattern of thoughts and nonthoughts.

Stability and Change. The idea that people select their environments is a useful way of thinking about how it is we sometimes change, and sometimes stay the same. By and large, most social theorists argue that the choice of our surroundings helps us to stay the same. Sociologists have spoken of the "opportunity structures" we build for ourselves that channel our subsequent behaviors in directions consistent with our past lives.[83] Social psychologists concerned with how people think about themselves have noted that we tend to seek situations that will promote the verification of our prior views of who we are.[84] Clinical psychologists have noted that we seek situations that perpetuate our prior moods.[85] And personality psychologists have stressed, too, that we commonly seek out circumstances that allow the expression of our personality characteristics.[86]

It makes sense that these psychological "nests" we build for ourselves would usually promote continuity. Each reminder we collect to cue a thought in the future, each one we discard to eliminate a thought in the future, is a bridge between our current selves and what we wish to be later on.[87] This psychological nest-building process gives us a comfortable place to think tomorrow, and tends to keep us thinking along the same lines from one day to the next. It is only fair to mention, however, that this process holds the potential to constrict our thoughts, limit our horizons, and keep us making the same errors over and over. If we are currently being wrongheaded about something, then setting up our lives in favor of continuity will keep us thinking wrongheaded thoughts and avoiding right-headed ones well into the future.

Eventually, we may realize this. Some unwanted thought may sneak in and undermine our whole system of wrongheadedness. We suddenly learn that our past and present way of thinking and acting is a failure, an inadequate response in some way to the unwanted thought before us. A clear example of this is the case of conversion. When people make a conversion, they appear to experience a thoroughgoing, radical revision of their way of understanding themselves and their worlds.[88] Thoughts that were previously unwanted can become wanted, and thoughts previously wanted can no longer be tolerated.

There are many kinds of conversion. Most quickly brought to mind is the religious variety, and this is certainly a clear example of a major life change. People also experience political conversions, as when Arthur Koestler became a Communist in 1931 and wrote ". . . something had clicked in my brain which shook me like a mental explosion. . . . The whole universe [fell] into a pattern like the stray pieces of a jigsaw puzzle assembled by magic at one stroke."[89] There are also personal conversions, resolutions to change that introduce major transformations of thought and behavior. The conversion from smoker to non-smoker, for example, can be a major life change that has many of the properties of a religious experience.

Facing up to an unwanted thought is usually the beginning. Some thought you have been fighting for some time finally breaks into consciousness, often prompted by an event that makes this unavoidable. You attend a religious meeting and are reminded of your current unhappiness or guilt; you go to the doctor and learn that your cholesterol intake is so high that heart disease is a clear danger; you are told by your partner that your constant jealousy is just insane, and that the relationship is in peril; you read a book that starts out innocently and eventually turns into a graphic reminder of your disturbing racist tendencies. With the unwanted thought exposed, you then see a solution—salvation, a low-cholesterol diet, turning over a "new leaf" to stop being jealous, a change in your racial outlook. This solution will require more than the basic decision, of course, so you set off to begin your new life.

There is a common tendency to see conversions of every kind as somehow magical, as though leprechauns must play a major role in the process. In large part, this is because *successful* conversions are usually the only ones we hear about. When we see someone who has truly changed, we wonder at what could have caused such a metamorphosis. How many times, though, do people experience the first few mental steps toward a conversion, or even feel the full emotional impact of that first awakening—to Christ, to Karl Marx, to nonsmoking, to an exercise program, to no more drinking, or the like—and then have this remarkable transformation fall flat in a few days or weeks? There are many unsuccessful attempts to make major life changes, and only a few that surface over time as truly lasting instances of radical change.[90]

Those that do succeed usually do so with massive aid from external sources of thought control. Although any fresh convert will scoff at the idea that the change is soft, a will-o'-the-wisp that can easily disappear, this is closer to the truth than the convert's likely stories of newly forged resolve and iron determination. Conversions that work, it turns out, are almost always accompanied by significant changes in life situations, transformations in the circumstances of the convert that promote continued thinking in the new direction. The reformed smoker cannot continue to carry tobacco, keep ashtrays around, sit in the smoking section of a restaurant or aircraft, or even spend much time with people who still smoke without risking a return to the old ways. This is probably why reformed smokers are usually far more obnoxious to smokers than are people who never even started.

An intriguing illustration of the power of external control comes from the history of the Methodist Church.[91] John Wesley, its principal founder, was preaching in England and America at about the same time as George Whitefield, a man who preached as widely but who never led his converts to create a church. Wesley, it seems, was keenly aware of the need to follow up the initial conversion experiences prompted by his preaching with further social support. He formed societies following his campaigns, groups in which new converts could find friends, encouragement, and further instruction in their faith. Whitefield just preached, and in the end admitted: "My brother Wesley acted wisely. The souls that were awakened under his ministry he joined in class, and thus preserved the fruit of his labor. This I neglected, and my people are a rope of sand."[92]

The external cues to thought that we find in other people, as in places and things, are crucial for the maintenance of change. If we desire to be different, we must arrange our social and physical circumstances to aid our efforts. The remote control of thinking, in this light, becomes much more than a parlor illusion we sometimes perpetrate on ourselves. The provision of an environment for change is the cornerstone of any new life we are attempting to construct. Because our thoughts are so deeply implied by all the things around us, we must take care to arrange our surroundings to yield the thoughts we desire.

Although we have spoken of "environments" and "cues" for thought as though they were usually places or things, it is really the social environment that prompts our thoughts most often. We can change our thoughts or keep them the same, therefore, by the company we keep. When we choose someone to have as an intimate partner, for example, we can look forward to talking with this person a lot, perhaps forever. What our partner thinks will always be there to stimulate our thinking as well. This means that if we pick a partner who agrees with us, we will seldom be challenged to change. If we pick someone who disagrees, we will often be called upon to revise our opinions.

This is particularly notable when what our partners agree or disagree with us about is ourselves. Some people have partners who disagree with them about what they are like. The egotistical, know-it-all husband whose wife thinks he is really a schmuck is an example. So, too, is the meek and self-effacing wife whose husband says she is the hardheaded boss of the household. In these cases a partner has a view of the person that is incongruent with the person's self-view. Partners can also have views of us that are congruent with what we think of ourselves.

Partners who have congruent views of us will help to protect us from information that might make us change. In one experiment, people who believed that they were socially anxious were given a psychological test and afterwards were told that they were not anxious at all—and instead appeared to handle social interaction in a graceful and competent manner.[93] This feedback is, of course, inconsistent with what they thought about themselves, and one might think that it would lead them to change their self-views somewhat. This is indeed what happened among those who were allowed after getting the feedback to chat with their partner—and whose partners' views of them happened to be incongruent with their views of themselves. Among those participants whose partners' views of them were congruent with their views of themselves, however, the chat led them to reject the feedback and return to their view of themselves as socially anxious.

A parallel pattern was observed among those individuals who believed at the outset that they were not anxious but received feedback that they were. They came to agree with this feedback if they had a chance to discuss it with a partner who also thought they were anxious, and to disagree with it if they talked with a partner who believed they were not anxious. Talking with one's partner can promote either change or stability in one's self-conception, depending on the partner's view of what one is like. We often may choose our partners, like we choose other features of our lives, as a way of promoting the stability or the change we desire.

Contexts for Suppression. People may underestimate the power that situations have on their thinking.[94] This means that the use of remote control processes is probably only a rudimentary skill for most of us, an ability we use once in a while and not always very well. The enterprise of remote control is complicated further by a surprising effect of thought suppression: Trying not to think about something in a particular context can make that context likely later to remind us of the very thought we were trying to suppress.

Recall the process of self-distraction. As noted earlier, the usual response to an unwanted thought is a series of attempts to distract ourselves. We enlist whatever we can find to think about in an effort to replace the unwanted thought with something more interesting. Now, where are these distracters likely to come from? Right, they are usually the handiest thoughts we can find—the ones prompted by our current surroundings. On trying not to think of having another piece of pie at Grandma's house, we look at her, we glance at the doilies on the furniture, we stare at her silly old dog, and perhaps we eventually succeed in suppressing the thought of the pie. What, then, are we inclined to be reminded of whenever we think of a doily? Maybe Grandma, maybe the dog—or maybe pie.

The situations in which we suppress a thought can become, over time, robust cues to the thought we wished to abandon there. Because we usually distract ourselves from unwanted thoughts in an unfocused way, ranging over many different replacement thoughts, the replacements we find in our current context can make that context a cue to the unwanted thought. The case of one gentleman who quit smoking in the hospital is relevant. He was in the hospital for a stomach problem unrelated to the smoking, but took the opportunity of being ill to quit. Now, several years since the successful abandonment of unwanted thoughts of cigarettes, he reports that a recent visit to that hospital produced the most thoughts of smoking, and the greatest urge, he has experienced since the original cold turkey days.

There is experimental evidence indicating that our surroundings can indeed become "spoiled" by suppression. A study was conducted in which people were asked to avoid thinking of a white bear while they reported everything that crossed their minds, and the effects of this suppression on their subsequent thinking in that context were investigated.[95] As in the original white bear study, participants were invited after the initial suppression task to continue reporting whatever came to mind, but now to *try* to think of a white bear. Remember that this opportunity to think about the white bear following suppression usually results in a special preoccupation with white bear, a "rebound" of thinking as compared to the thought frequency of people who are asked only to think about white bear from the outset.

All participants in this new experiment viewed a slide show as they suppressed and then subsequently expressed the white bear thought. For some participants, this slide show was designed to provide a constant context—they saw slides on one theme, such as "classroom scenes." For other participants, however, the slide show was arranged to introduce a new context between the suppression and expression periods. Here, slides of classrooms during suppression were replaced by slides of household appliances during later expression.

It makes sense, of course, that subjects whose context stayed constant would show the usual rebound of white bear thoughts during the expression period, as their experience was much like that of subjects in the original white bear study. And this is what happened; white bear thoughts among subjects in the "old context" increased over the five-minute period (their bell rings signaling the occurrence of the thought are shown in Figure 2). The subjects in the "new context" group, by comparison, were relieved of the usual rebound effect. Although subjects in this group might well have used the slides as self-distracters during suppression of white bear, these cues were removed when they later had the chance to think about white bear. During the expression opportunity, they were in a different psychological environment—a new set of slides—and so there were no reminders left from the earlier self-distraction to cue the continued return to white bear thoughts.

These findings suggest interesting possibilities. They imply, for instance, why "fat farms," "alcohol detox centers," "drug treatment centers," or other residential facilities for self-control problems may be so successful as compared to self-treatment at

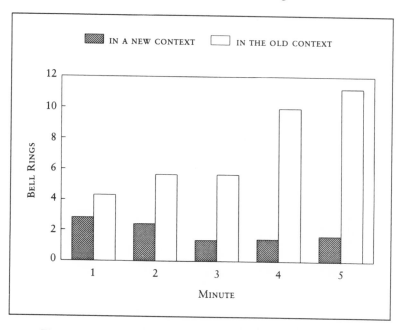

Figure 2. EXPRESSION OF WHITE BEAR THOUGHTS
FOLLOWING SUPPRESSION

home. Of course, having lots of people around who expect you to control yourself is an important start, and the locked doors don't hurt either; the external control is the first effect of this environment on suppression. But when people come home from such a place, they may benefit in addition from the fact that they have left the reminders of their addiction behind. Most of their self-distracters, the things they thought about in the attempt not to think of food, alcohol, their drug, or whatever addictive substance, are still back at the residential facility. And they are now home, with fewer cues to induce them into a relapse.

Of course, there are still reminders of the problem at home. These are not suppression-produced cues, though, merely the usual things that are associated with the unwanted thought. Say, the liquor cabinet is still there for the recovering alcoholic, even though the liquor may be removed. These reminders can be eliminated, too, with a careful job of remote control. But the great advantage of having suppressed elsewhere is that at home, things like the doorknob and the television and the bathroom tiles will not be as likely to serve as reminders of a drink. If one had tried to get on the wagon at home, one might have looked at and thought about all these things in the attempt to suppress the thought of alcohol. Enough mental exploration of the place in this self-distraction mind-set could have made almost everything a grim reminder of exactly what one did not want to consider.

With this perspective on unwanted thoughts, we can now see that there is good reason to play tricks on ourselves. We can't be perfectly direct and straightforward in the attempt to suppress an unwanted thought or desire, as we could promptly fail. We must enlist our circumstances to help us. For one, we should be sure to suppress in an environment that is not like the one in which we will later relax the suppression. And then, we should attempt to surround ourselves with people, places, and things that will help us hold on to our newfound freedom from the unwanted thought. We must assemble around us people who agree with our new viewpoint; we must go to places that will allow us to see and hear what we want to hold in consciousness; we must retain those objects that remind us of what we truly wish to think. All this sounds like a tremendous lot of trouble, and it is. We can certainly foul up our present circumstances, perhaps permanently, in doing what seems to be nothing but arranging our future thoughts. But we need help when we set out to control our minds, and the best help we can get is through remote control—changing the world that our minds think about.

SIX

The Will
to Disbelieve

*An image-proposition is necessarily positive: we can imagine
the window to the left of the door, or to the right of the door,
but we can form no image of the bare negative "the window
not to the left of the door." We can disbelieve the image-
proposition expressed by "the window to the left of the door,"
and our disbelief will be true if the window is not to the left
of the door. But we can form no image of the fact that the
window is not to the left of the door.*

—Bertrand Russell, *The Analysis of Mind*

In a court of law, it sometimes happens that something will
slip out that could unfairly influence the jury's verdict. This
information is judged to have an improper influence, though,
and so someone tries to "take it back." The judge may ask the
jury to disregard what one of the attorneys said, for example,
or an attorney may ask the judge to have some testimony a
witness has volunteered stricken from the record. When this
happens, justice proceeds blindly while everyone else in the
courtroom rolls their eyes—realizing that information that is
"taken back" in this way never truly disappears. Although legal
arguments often hinge on the assumption that people can
disregard a thought or remove it from consideration in making
a decision, this nonetheless seems very hard to do.

Now, there are many reasons to suspect that we do have some
willful control over how we use information. William James

wrote in *The Will to Believe,* for instance, that the desire to believe something could create belief.[96] He was stating the case for religious faith, belief built not on knowledge but on need. There are instances in which just such belief can be demonstrated, and there is good reason to think that people's desires can indeed mold much of their view of what is true.[97] Exceptions to this rule do exist, though, particularly in instances when we wish to disbelieve something or disregard its implications for our beliefs.

The topic of this chapter is how thoughts that we cannot erase from our mind continue to influence our further thinking. The chapter thus represents something of a turning point in the flow of the book—from a concern with how mental control works to a focus on what effect mental control can have. We will begin by considering some key examples, cases in which it appears that people are led to make faulty judgments because they cannot disregard information that is available to them. The question of how disbelief and disregard operate is taken up next. We will develop a view of these matters that allows us to understand when people will fail to ignore thoughts, and when they will succeed in ignoring them. As we shall soon learn, the failure to ignore is most striking when people have little information on which to base their judgments.

Incrimination Through Innuendo. What happens when, in the grocery checkout line, you glance over to a tabloid and read the headline MOTHER STABS SON WITH FORK? This idea reverberates through your mind to create a special niche, a bizarre image. Suppose, however, that you read a story later in which this headline is fully retracted, the cruel hoax is uncovered, and photos are shown of the happy mom and son with no eating utensils anywhere in view. Does this new story truly remove the initial impression? It certainly does not erase it. We know from the white bear studies that it takes much more than a retraction to produce a lasting and effective suppression. So, the effect of seeing a headline and retraction is that you now know *two* things—the headline and the retraction. You may use them to reach some overall judgment about what happened, a judgment that may draw on both ideas. But the headline does not go away.

This fact is often used by news reporters. What they do is report their news in a form that already contains some sort of "retraction"—a hedge or qualification that recommends readers take the news with a grain of salt. So, for instance, in a television story about a physician accused of intentionally poisoning his patients, Barbara Walters concluded by asking: "Would you let this man give you an aspirin?" This innuendo is legally safer than saying the physician is a poisoner, of course, because it is phrased as a question. Yet the message seems to get across. By the time Barbara was done, most viewers would probably not even give the man an aspirin.

In a study of innuendo effects, my students and I gave people an innuendo headline to read.[98] We told them that they were reading about a candidate for a city council election in another city. The headline was: IS BOB TALBERT LINKED WITH MAFIA? After this, they were asked to report their evaluation of Bob Talbert by rating him on a series of dimensions (for example, honest vs. dishonest, pleasant vs. unpleasant). It was found that the question about his link with the Mafia made these students view him negatively. They saw him as much less admirable than did students who read only an innocuous headline (BOB TALBERT ARRIVES IN CITY). Moreover, their impressions of him were almost exactly as negative as those reached by students who read a directly incriminating assertion (BOB TALBERT LINKED WITH MAFIA). Although questions may represent little more than "fishing expeditions," they can be every bit as incriminating as direct statements.

So far, this study seems just to confirm what many of us already suspected about the nature of media innuendo. When a possibility is raised by a headline or story, especially one that was not previously considered by readers, it can be very persuasive. Eyebrows go up, glances are exchanged, and there is a collective murmur of recognition. Politicians seem always to be chastising the press for just this kind of reporting. The appropriate reparation in these cases is clear: The press must be called upon to deny or retract such false suggestions, right?

The hopes we might hold for such a solution are dimmed considerably, though, by one other finding of this innuendo study. The study also tested reactions to another kind of headline, the denial. A different group of students read only this: BOB TALBERT NOT LINKED WITH MAFIA. These students turned out to be not quite so negative toward Bob Talbert as those who read the question headline (IS BOB . . . ?) or the direct assertion (BOB IS . . .). However, they were still much more negative than those who read the innocuous statement. In short, saying Talbert was not linked with Mafia made people dislike him. Rather than a denial removing or neutralizing the incrimination, and thus acting as one expects denials to act, here it *caused* incrimination.

But don't blame this all on the press. Admittedly, their use of innuendo and even of denial does help them convey news. Reporters must walk a thin line between writing what is already known (and so is boring) and what is only suspected (and thus exciting but potentially false and libelous). Innuendo aids in the communication of such information, because it combines the new and interesting with the sober qualification. Therefore, the media use this form of communication frequently. They did not, however, invent it. Everyone finds it useful, at some point, to say something and appear to take it back at the same time.[99] Innuendos are part of the human communicative apparatus, always present, sometimes used effectively, and sometimes fallen into like an open manhole. A former president of the U.S., after all, committed one of the finest self-innuendos of all time when he said "I am not a crook." A triple gainer into a manhole if ever there was one.

The power of innuendo comes from the fact that the ideas

we communicate may be difficult to disbelieve or disregard at will. Innuendo occurs when we communicate disavowal along with our ideas. We attach comments that are meant, at least on the surface, to qualify, question, deny, or even apologize. Jimmy Carter, for instance, carried forward his second presidential campaign by noting that he would not crack under pressure—and that this comment was not meant to refer to Teddy Kennedy's performance at Chappaquiddick. In another interesting case, this one a controversy over the refurbishing of the Statue of Liberty, then President Reagan's chief of staff Donald Regan was quoted in *Time* as saying "I do not hate Lee Iacocca's guts." Obviously, the ideas are there no matter what gets added. Just *mentioning* something is enough to guarantee that the minds of those who hear it will never be the same.

False Feedback.   In the sixties, a psychologist gave some men a personality test and reported to them afterwards that they were "latent homosexuals."[100] This was part of a scientific study, so the men were at least startled and probably quite shaken. The psychologist, however, was lying. His story was designed to induce "lowered self-esteem" in these men for the purpose of testing their later reactions. And, of course, the men were informed after the study that the test results had been false.

Naturally, this study and ones like it raised quite a furor in the field. Are the aims of psychologists so wonderful that they justify putting people through this sort of mental anguish? Even though the psychologist's lies are eventually revealed, there is a period of time during which the research participants truly believe they are something they are not. Needless to say, research of this kind is reviewed very carefully these days, and is conducted only when it is clear to many people (including government-sanctioned review boards) that the potential benefits outweigh the potential costs. Deceit is still sometimes used in such research, however, and the nagging question that remains is whether, when people are "debriefed" about such lies, they come back to normal.

Researchers have tested whether experimental deceptions can be erased, and the findings are worrisome.[101] In one study, for instance, participants were asked to perform the task of judging which of a pair of suicide notes came from an actual suicide victim.[102] In the process of judging a long series of these pairs, some participants were told that they did very well, whereas others were told that they did not do well. This "false feedback" was simply up to chance—the experimenter determined by a random drawing whether subjects would be told they succeeded or failed. After this, some of the participants were informed that the feedback had been false. The ruse and the random drawing were completely revealed. When asked to predict how they would do on this task if they tried it again, though, these people still showed effects of the feedback. They expected to succeed if their false feedback had indicated success, and to fail if their false feedback had indicated failure—even though they were informed that the feedback had been fiction.

People watching all this were similarly affected. When some participants were assigned only to *observe* the goings-on, and then were informed, just as were the participants themselves, that the feedback was false, they trusted the feedback as a guide to how the participants would do on the task in the future. Even though observers were "dehoaxed," they continued to believe that the people in the study were the kind of people who deserve the feedback they were given.

Innuendo and false feedback seem to have something in common. In both cases, people learn something that is revealed as untrue. With innuendo, they learn, for example, that someone in the news is a criminal—but that this may not be true. People in false feedback studies learn that someone has succeeded or failed at a task—and then find out later that this is not true. If the influence of innuendo and false feedback come from the same psychological process, we can make an additional prediction: We would expect that it doesn't matter *when* people are issued the denial in a false feedback study. After all, innuendos are powerful even though the denial of the underlying information is offered at the very same time as the information— as in ROY DID NOT HOLD UP THE FILLING STATION. This statement, at face value, indicates that Roy is innocent. But of course, we know there must be something wrong with him, don't we? Even the denial that is communicated with the incriminating information fails to disabuse us of our inevitably negative impression.

This reasoning leads to the idea that people in psychological experiments might not even respond properly to a *briefing*—a revelation at the beginning of the experiment that the feedback they are to receive will be false. This was tested in research that repeated all the essential features of the earlier false feedback studies.[103] Participants in this new experiment, however, were told *in advance* of performing the suicide note judgment task that the feedback they were to receive would be false. And these participants then went through the entire procedure, making discriminations between notes, hearing the feedback, and so on, one pair of notes at a time through 25 pairs. A succession of observers participated also, each watching a different participant go through the task.

Then, the key question was asked. Both participants and observers were asked how the participant would do on an upcoming genuine judgment task of the same kind. Now remember, these people were *forewarned* that everything they would see in the study would be a sham. And yet, the majority fell for the false feedback. Experiencing false success led both participants and observers to believe that the participant would continue to succeed; and experiencing false failure led them to believe that the participant would continue to fail. Whether we learn before, during, or after we encounter a piece of information that the information is false, we may subsequently use the information in just the same way. We embrace the information, hold it fondly, and fail to ignore it when we rightfully should. Remember, the success or failure that was observed in these studies was made up in advance, play-acted by the experimenter, had no connection to real events, and by literary standards was not even very good fiction. It was nothing at all. But people remembered it, and when the time came to make a judgment, they used it.

Let's take a brief moment to reflect on professional wrestling. Remember last weekend (pick any weekend) when Rocko "Cement Truck" Brewster destroyed his opponent with a flying elbow drop? The announcer reminded us that "there's no escape from that flying elbow drop. It's curtains for sure." Rocko threatened to attack the TV camera as he left the ring, of course, and then it was over. We don't really *believe* all this, do we? We have known since junior high school that wrestling is staged, just like roller derby, and that no one ever really gets hurt or wins or loses in these matches. But then there's that sensational flying elbow drop. Rocko stands atop the corner ropes high above his opponent, and then falls through the air, driving that elbow sharply against the gentleman's chest. Or at least, so it *seems*.

This is false feedback, too. Lies. But that really doesn't seem to matter in our experience of the event, and given the chance we would probably vote for Rocko in any upcoming bout, even a real one. Why? What is it about some thoughts that makes them so "sticky," so difficult to ignore when it comes time to decide what is true and false, what matters and what doesn't? The media innuendos, the false feedback in experiments, and the professional wrestling shows all share a special quality that seems to thwart the will to disbelieve, an irresistible force that persuades us even in the face of the seemingly immovable object of falsity.

The Next Thought.   One way to understand the irresistible force of false ideas is to consider where they lead us. What do we typically think *next*, after we have just encountered an idea and its denial? Suppose we hear, for instance, that Millie is "not fat." If this denial (*not fat*) leads us to think of the underlying idea that has been denied (*fat*), and it does this more quickly and directly than it leads us to think of things that are consistent with the denial itself (she is *thin*), then it will usually have the tendency to maintain the truth of the denied idea in our minds (this woman is huge). If, however, a denial leads us to think of things that follow from the denial (*thinness*) rather than from the underlying denied information (all that *fat*), then we will be able to reason in the logical way—accepting a denial as a statement that makes something false (she is indeed *not* fat).

Consider your cousin Lloyd the hypochondriac. He has been to three doctors in the past six months, complaining to all of them about dizziness and headaches. They X-rayed his head, did blood tests, and even a CAT scan, and in the end, they reported that there was nothing physically wrong. There was no brain tumor. This denial, you would think, would lead him quickly to think about other things. Freed of a potential problem, he should be thinking about playing tennis, or having sex, or taking up some other vice that deathly ill people envy. But instead, when he thinks of the doctors' verdict, he is no doubt reminded of the brain tumor. "My brain is not turning to mush in my head, not being pressed out my ears by a tumor, not having a stroke, not riddled with foreign growths," he says to himself. The denials continue to remind him first of the symptoms of illness, and perhaps only later of what he now might do if the denials are true—so, the denials do not work.

As long as a falsification reminds us more quickly of what it is not rather than what it is, it will fail. If "There will be no earthquake in Los Angeles," for instance, leads L.A. residents to think about whether their homes will withstand an earthquake, rather than about the weather or what to do this Saturday, then it will be a useless denial, a falsification that does more damage than good. The next thought we think after a denial or an admonishment to disregard something, then, is a key to whether these things will operate as advertised. If a denial can redirect attention away from the denied information, and toward something else that is consistent with the denial, then it will work.

This is what happens in the many instances in which people do appear to ignore false information. Certainly, when someone is accused of murder but is found innocent, we do not then put the person to death. True, we may still make the person pay, perhaps dearly, for having been so accused. The information that the person was NOT A MURDERER lives on, just as do all denials. But we *are* capable of understanding the meaning of denial to some degree, at least to the point that we can often respond appropriately to the realization that something is false. The accused murderer found innocent is set free, usually because the judge and jury are no longer dwelling on the negative, the idea that this person is not a murderer, but rather have moved to think about what else is true in light of this. They have a theory of what happened, and this alternative body of ideas allows the "murderer" thought to be defused by the denial.

The question, then, becomes a matter of *when*. When does a denial (not-A) lead people to continue thinking of the underlying information (A), or to move to thoughts of information consistent with the denial (B, a fact that follows from not-A)? The answer can be understood by analyzing some of the examples we have already discussed. In the case of Roy, the fellow who did not hold up the filling station, we are clearly in the presence of a thought that is hard to disbelieve. No matter how much we rail about his innocence, no matter how loud this denial may become, Roy is still left with a bad reputation. This is because *we know nothing else about him,* about the filling station, or about this entire episode. Quite simply, we are information-starved, and anyone who asks us about Roy is bound to hear our only tidbit of gossip, meager as it is.

"Know anything about Roy?" they ask, testing whether we've been awake.

"Didn't hold up the filling station," we reply, proud to have this fact.

"Is he a bad boy?" they now wonder.

"Can't say," we say. And everyone goes home with a bad opinion of Roy, ready to hide the silver if he ever comes to visit.

When we have an impoverished store of information on any topic, ideas about that topic will be difficult to disbelieve. This was certainly the case in most of the research we have discussed to this point. The innuendo headlines, surely, were about people whom no one knows. (Bob Talbert, despite all his sins, was only a fictional character.) And the false feedback studies, likewise, asked people to judge someone's upcoming performance on a suicide note judgment task. It is not as though the average person turns to the morning paper and, after completing the crossword, gamely tackles the suicide note discrimination page. This is a downright odd thing to do, a task for which people have only little relevant information. Thus, when they receive even wholly false information, the denial of the information turns out to be ineffective. Nothing else about a person's likelihood of success at such a task is known, so people grasp at straws—the ideas that are false but relevant.

This suggests a further observation: The will to disbelieve cannot make a thought irrelevant to another thought. Thoughts we wish to disbelieve remain available to us, and are especially likely to be drawn from when we have *nothing else on which to depend*. So, for example, reconsider the man who is NOT A MURDERER. If we knew nothing else of him, he might be in big trouble. Imagine meeting a stranger who was wearing a sign with this legend. Would you invite him into your home? Introduce him to your loved ones? Ask him to hand you a knife? You might not put him to death, but you probably would banish him from your life. And if you were society as a whole, that would amount to a life sentence for him.

Only if you knew that this person also wore a red suit, had several reindeer, and shook when he laughed like a bowl full of jelly, would the stigma of his sign begin to fade. This is SANTA! And just think—you almost banished him from your house forever, for *not* being a murderer. With no other information on which to base your judgment, you used the only idea you had. The thought was not made irrelevant by disbelief, and it was therefore available for use in the absence of anything better. Now that we know who this is, we have much more relevant information on which to base judgments of this person.

The danger of ignorance now becomes apparent. When we know little relevant to a judgment we must make, we will turn to nonfacts, ideas that stick in our minds but are demonstrably wrong. So, for instance, someone who is ignorant about football watching is not just a novice about plays, about players, or about how the game proceeds. Such a person is also unlikely to be able to entertain the idea that one team in a game will win without coming to believe that this outcome is inevitable.[104] The novice has no other ideas about how things may come out, and these other ideas would be important help in the enterprise of ignoring the imaginary and false outcome that is the only one being "considered." People who are not expert become swayed toward thinking one team must win after they just think about why that might happen. Given one scenario for thinking that Michigan State will beat Notre Dame (for instance, that their backfield is very, very fast), the novice football fan may well come to expect that the Spartans of MSU will prevail. The expert can generate other scenarios and so is not overwhelmed by this one.[105]

The same kind of thing happens when we meet someone new for the first time. If we are told this person is likely to be an introvert, we will usually go about asking questions that presuppose the person is shy. We might ask the stranger if he or she had ever spent an evening at a party sitting in a closet. If we are told the person may be an extrovert, however, our line of questioning changes. The next thing we will think is usually going to be related to extroversion—so we might ask this person if he or she enjoyed speaking extemporaneously to a group. But if we are told the person is *not an introvert,* we will make the odd move of asking questions about the person's degree of introversion. Rather than transforming this idea in our minds, making "not introvert" into "extrovert," we simply strip away the denial and work directly with the underlying information. In meeting strangers, we take any information we get as our cue for what to think next—even when that information is hidden under a direct attempt at falsification.[106]

It appears, then, that we can be lazy in our attempts to think the right thing, make the proper judgment. When we know little else, we take the idea we have (even if it is marked as false), and track it down to the next idea in line. That next idea is very likely to depend on exactly how the first idea is phrased in our minds. If we hear "not bad," we think "bad" next; if we hear "bad," we also do this. If we hear "not good," though, we will think next of "good," just as though we had heard "good" from the start.

The Problem of Ignorance. Ignorance creates the "weakness" in our will to disbelieve. Like a still pool in which a single pebble's entrance yields many ripples, a mind that is empty will be notably perturbed by a single idea, even when that idea is hypothetical or false. The problem seems to be that a thought in isolation yields two mental possibilities—the thought and its opposite. When these are all we know, there is little to decide between them. They form a channel of thought, a pair of possibilities that are mutually exclusive, yet somehow bound up together.

This property of thoughts is illustrated by the reversible figure shown in box (a) in Figure 3. This is a drawing of a Necker Cube, an oddity noted by perception psychologists that you may have produced many times in your own doodles without knowing its name. The cube has the property of *reversible perspective.* When you look at it, you may see the lower face forward—the one shown shaded in box (b); or you may see the upper face

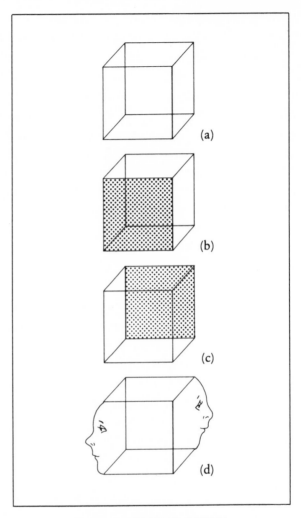

Figure 3. NECKER CUBES

forward—the one shaded in box (c). You can reverse this figure in your mind's eye, changing from one perspective to the other. Some people find the last version (d) easiest to reverse, making each face come to the front in turn.

Thoughts present more than one perspective to us in just this way. Each thought we entertain suggests both its truth and its falsity, its positive and its negative aspect, its reality and its fantasy. When we look at it, it can reverse itself in our mind. The WRESTLING CHAMP is linked with the NOT WRESTLING CHAMP, and vice versa; the NOT A MURDERER is linked with A MURDERER, and vice versa. Each thought travels in our minds with its denial, offering us both possibilities whenever we encounter just one. Although we may become convinced that just one perspective on the thought is correct, and may see it that way each time we consider it on many consecutive occasions, the opposite possibility is always nearby, contained in our mental representation of the thought itself, and so ready to jump out and impress us with no notice at all.

This means that each thought we encounter can be represented as a whole cube. It is not only a thought, but contains the seed of its opposite as well. Once the whole cube is presented to us, there is nothing we can do short of full-blown attempts at suppression that will make it go away. Once we have said "Your hair doesn't look so bad this way," the cat is out of the bag and it cannot be put back inside. We can attempt to promote the opposite view of the thought we have let slip, as we then apologize—sometimes for months—about our awkward hair compliment. Having put the remark as a denial of badness, we are now stuck with the "could be bad" side of the cube facing out, perhaps more often than the "not bad" side. Suggesting that the thought is wrong or false or silly or mistaken will not make it truly disappear.

Only when a thought is brought into the context of other thoughts does it begin to stabilize, presenting a consistent aspect to us each time we consider it. This is illustrated with the additional Necker Cube shown in Figure 4. This one has all the same features as a completely reversible cube, but because of its context, tends to present only one aspect of itself to us. Certainly, the practiced perceiver can still reverse even this with

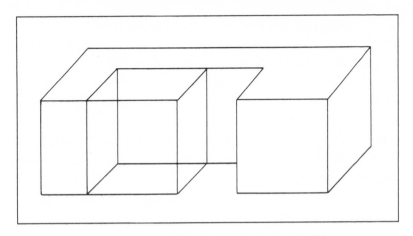

Figure 4. NECKER CUBE IN CONTEXT

little difficulty. But the context suggests quite strongly that the cube should be seen in just one way, and we usually see it that way.

In the context of other thoughts, then, a thought will hold still. It will be either true to us or false to us, and we will tend not to notice the opposite. The context of other thoughts is either consistent with the thought (one perspective) or consistent with its denial (the other perspective) and so inclines us toward accepting either the thought or its denial, but not both. In the case of the backhanded compliment about our friend's hair being "not so bad," we can help to promote the more flattering interpretation of what we said by purchasing our friend a gift, making additional (proper) compliments, or asking if our friend is considering becoming a professional model. The interpretation of a thought and its opposite begins to stabilize in one direction only when we have many thoughts that stand together to yield a consistent picture. Even then, of course, the original thought is still impossible to suppress. The cube will not go away; all we can do is reverse it.

This framework for understanding belief and disbelief emphasizes the "qualitative" side of mental life. We too often view the human mind in a "quantitative" or graduated way, believing that we can understand thought as occurring in continuous increments, shades of difference along some dimension. For example, we speak of our attitude toward a political candidate as a matter of *degree*—how much do we like the candidate? Similarly, we may seek to determine how sad or how happy a person is, how much the person expects rain, or how deeply the person believes in ESP. And usually, we would be happy to learn the person's answers by seeing what point the person checks along some gradual scale—for example, from 1 to 10, "strongly agree" to "strongly disagree." Each question assumes that beliefs or attitudes are matters of degree.

This assumption obscures an important fact about the mind: There is a greater mental leap between ignorance and knowledge than the distance separating the gradations between different sorts of knowledge. When the person learns of the political candidate in the first place, discovers an emotion of happiness or sadness, learns that rain is possible, or realizes that ESP is something to consider, the jump from ignorance to knowledge has been made. This is a *qualitative* change, a movement from mental nothing to mental something. In a sense, it is the creation of the entire Necker Cube. And this transition is far more important for all of thinking than any of the various quantitative changes our mind experiences.

Denial, disbelief, and disregard work as though they were quantitative changes. To say "I will not commit suicide," for instance, is a denial. This thought is the opposite of "I will commit suicide." As such, it is only a statement of how much suicide it is good to have. The denial presupposes the idea of suicide itself. Thus, a qualitative leap—from not knowing about suicide as a possibility to thinking of it as possible—is included as a hidden part of a quantitative statement. The entire Necker Cube comes along when we want to convey only one perspective. This may be why suicide seems contagious. It could explain why three students at Bryan High School on the outskirts of

Omaha, Nebraska, committed suicide within five days, and why an additional four of their classmates made attempts within three weeks. Once the possibility of suicide is brought to mind, even amid exclamations of genuine horror and dismay, it becomes a part of the mind, a mental quality. Expressions of shock and admonitions *not* to commit suicide amount only to quantitative variations on the original theme.

When we have an idea that is well worth erasing, one that just cries out to be wiped off the face of the earth, the most direct attack we can imagine making on it is to say it is false. The fact that disbelieved ideas do not "go away," however, leaves us with this potentially tricky, oscillating idea in our mind. Sometimes we will remember it is false, and we will make decisions accordingly. But at other times we may lose track of our disbelief, or our resolution to disregard this idea, and so make judgments that follow from the belief that the thought is true. All we really have to go on, though, is that the thought exists in our mind.[107]

Turn back now to the problem of evidence that a jury is instructed to disregard in court. The instruction cannot produce an erasure, a complete suppression. So, what is left is a remarkably volatile mental state. The jurors have the information, and the degree to which they use it or avoid it will be entirely dependent on how well they *remember to disbelieve*. If they are constantly on watch, and have enough additional facts to make sense of the case without the to-be-disregarded information, they may get by without ever using the forbidden ideas. If they just once forget to disbelieve, however, especially in the face of little additional knowledge, the forbidden ideas may very well surface and influence their judgments. If you were on trial, would you want to trust their vigilance?

We must recognize that any admonitions to disbelieve, deny, or disregard a thought are generally "extra baggage" in our minds. Our thinking processes appear to deal most quickly and efficiently with positive instances ("It is red") rather than negative ones ("It is not green"). This tendency is so strong that we usually seem to translate negatives into positives in our mind whenever we can.[108] Dealing with double and triple negatives becomes completely impossible, and we do what we can to avoid them—in good prose and in our mind as well. The work of interpreting and remembering those pesky denials is probably, in the end, what makes thoughts so very difficult to disregard. The denial has to be dragged along, like an unruly child, wherever the family of thought decides to visit. If it runs off or hides under the table, we will mistake the thought for truth in the meantime. In essence, disbelief is a two-step process, acceptance followed by denial, and when the second step fails we are left with the products of the first.[109]

The only way to counteract this is with more thoughts. With lots of consistent information available, we are reminded about the disregarding or disbelieving we must do. Thus, for instance, by this point in the chapter you've probably succeeded completely in disregarding the possibility raised earlier—that Santa Claus was a murderer. Even though the murderer—not a murderer dimension was brought up with regard to him, there is no effect of this. Although the will to disbelieve is not, by itself, sufficient to clear our minds of false thoughts or their unwanted implications, more knowledge of what is true can do it. To eradicate those ideas that we wished to clear from the jurors' minds, it will be necessary to come up with a *counterexplanation*—a full-blown story that accounts for the to-be-ignored ideas and makes them easy to ignore, in the light of other clarifying information.

Overcoming Prejudicial Beliefs. Racist, sexist, and other prejudiced ideas often arrive in the form of denials and calls to disbelieve. We learn that women are no longer mere housewives, that Jews are not unusually rich, that blacks and Hispanics are not any more prone to crime than people of other groups when their relative poverty is taken into account, that monogamous gay males are no more likely than heterosexual males to be carriers of AIDS . . . and so on, in a series of refutations of our potential prejudices. Can we reject our stereotypical beliefs when we learn these things? It would seem that the same processes underlying the acceptance of innuendo and the failure to reject false feedback would be in operation here—with the unfortunate result that prejudices are perpetuated even when we try to reject them.

Dealing with our prejudices can be complicated. At times we can accept unfair stereotypes completely, tell racial jokes or laugh at them, avoid people whose race or ethnic group is different from our own, and perhaps even do what we can to hurt them. At the very least, we may curse under our breath at the rude person on the subway or the unobservant driver who made us swerve, incorporating the person's race into our unsaid insult and making a mental note that these people always do these kinds of things. At other times, however, we feel ashamed of our unfairness and we try to hide our beliefs. Certainly, we are careful to say something like "I'm not prejudiced, but . . ." before we reveal anything that remotely resembles a prejudiced observation.[110] We may even pretend never to have had a prejudiced thought in our lives. Ultimately, we will probably vacillate between these extremes and spend much of our time with the conflicting sides of our mind in an uneasy truce.

The difficulty, of course, is that we are caught between two forces. Our stereotypes are potentially useful generalizations about people, but they expose us to the ethical dilemma of treating individuals on the basis of false and unfair ideas. To be able to say something about a whole group of people at once is, after all, a great labor-saving device. It is better for an English-speaker to know that he or she will not be able to communicate with just about everyone in Japan, for instance, than it is for this person to walk around asking every individual the same question (Speak English? Speak English? Speak English?). And it is also true that generalizations about people can be dangerous and criminal. After all, it was a generalization that led to the slavery of blacks in America, another that instigated the mass murder of millions of Jews and other "undesirables" by the Nazis during World War II, and still others that even now promote continued injustices toward people in disadvantaged positions all over the world.

Each individual must choose, then, which generalizations are needed and should be believed—and which are likely to be morally harmful and should thus be questioned and regarded skeptically. The key to fighting the generalizations that are unfair, of course, is the same key we have identified in the fight against innuendo and other failures to deny. We need more information. As it turns out, people are often capable of disbelieving stereotyped information about someone when they are given sufficient "individuating" information to distinguish that person from the stereotyped group.[111] If we learn that Esteban is a medical student, for instance, it is comparatively easy to reject any stereotypical inferences about his habits, language, or abilities that might otherwise surface given only the knowledge of his Hispanic heritage. Without information about him as an individual, however, we are in the quandary of knowing only what it is prejudiced to believe.

The idea that people are ethically responsible for their beliefs is, in the end, an important source of moral guidance. We may not always be able to control our beliefs about others, for many of the cognitive processes by which we perceive people are automatic and beyond our control. And once formed, a false belief may be very difficult to reject. Yet the fact that we can intend to avoid prejudice, and on occasion can succeed in displacing our stereotyped inferences with real information about individuals, means that we can serve the goal of justice through mental control. If we seek always to learn more about others, to find out what individuals are like rather than jumping to conclusions based on their group memberships, we may overcome our tendencies to be prejudiced.

Can we exert a will to disbelieve? In this chapter, we have

seen that merely wanting to deny, to disbelieve, to falsify, is not enough. We cannot ignore information that is available to us, no matter how strong our wills. The key to disbelieving is having something to believe. If we wish to deny one idea, we must have another that we can put in its place.

SEVEN

Mood Control

To lift yourself out of a miserable mood, even if you have to do it by strength of will, should be easy. I force myself out of my chair, stride around the table, exercise my head and neck, make my eyes sparkle, tighten the muscles around them. Defy my own feelings, welcome A enthusiastically supposing he comes to see me, amiably tolerate B in my room, swallow all that is said at C's, whatever pain and trouble it may cost me, in long draughts.
Yet even if I manage that, one single slip, and a slip cannot be avoided, will stop the whole process, easy and painful alike, and I will have to shrink back into my own circle again.

—Franz Kafka, *Resolutions*

When I find myself feeling down, I usually respond in one of two ways. Sometimes I wallow in it. I put some blues on the stereo, sit still in my chair for a long while, and maybe fail to turn on the lights when the sun goes down. With the dusk glowing dully around furniture silhouettes, and B. B. King singing how nobody loves him but his mother, I get a pure form of despair, an unusual clarity of mind and mood that is somehow satisfying. I don't do this too often, though, because it can be frightening, almost hypnotic and overwhelming. The alternative is to thrash. I move against the feeling, working all the strategies I know of to propel myself into a better mood.

Thrashing may require going out to a movie, talking to someone, flipping through a magazine, having a cup of coffee or something to eat. Tammy Bakker, wife of the fallen TV evangelist Jim Bakker, recommends her own strategy in *Christian Wives:* "There's times I just have to quit thinking, and the only way I can quit thinking is by shopping." Thrashing may move other people to look at a travel brochure, to work on a hobby, or to review happy thoughts in their minds. The outcome of all this, however, can sometimes be deeply disappointing. The reason it seems more like "thrashing" than "escaping" is that we are frequently pulled right back into the negative mood. It is as though in thrashing we are trying to escape, but we don't know in quite what direction to go. So we try every one that comes to mind, and only on occasion do we get it right and get away.

This chapter is concerned with how we control our moods and emotions, particularly depressive ones. To start, we will explore some basic ideas about how moods operate, how they rule the coloration of our thoughts from moment to moment, and how thoughts themselves can give rise to moods. We will then investigate the results of a series of studies in which people were asked to attempt the suppression of mood-related thoughts. How can people think themselves out of bad moods? The solution, we shall find, is obvious: positive thinking. The problem, we shall learn, is that in the throes of depression, this solution can be exceptionally difficult to put into practice.

Emotion and Purpose. Psychology can claim few scientists who have won a Nobel prize, and Herbert Simon is one of them. He is also one of the originators of information processing psychology, the development of models of mind that draw from models of computation. One of Simon's many ideas is that smart machines must have both motivation and emotion.[112] He pointed out that a thinking machine would be stupid indeed if it did not possess these two important qualities, even though these qualities are ones that we human beings usually assume are very un-machinelike.

Motivation is important because it gives thinking a purpose.

Without a motive, an information processor would have no reason to pursue one line of processing to the exclusion of others. It could not be "single-minded," or develop priorities and so be able to think one thought until it is done and go on to the next. Emotion, on the other hand, is important for precisely the opposite reason. A thinking machine that is single-minded could, under the right conditions, keep working hard at calculating the value of pi to the millionth decimal, while a well-meaning but mistaken garden supply service was filling the room to the ceiling with peat moss. Emotion is needed to *break* purpose, to interrupt otherwise motivated thinking when prompt response to environmental demands is needed.[113]

In this way of understanding emotion, it is clear that emotion should not be very susceptible to willful control. If we could turn off all our emotions, feel no pain, never laugh, not be gripped by fear or despair, stop being excited, and so on, we could easily end up dead. Peat moss suffocation is not pretty. Emotions are built in by evolution, not to be tampered with, because hundreds of generations of humans before us have survived their friends or acquaintances who *were* able to shut down their emotions.[114] Disgust keeps us from eating icky things; sadness helps us notice our losses; fear reminds us to run from predators; joy keeps us coming back to our friends and sex partners. It is good, in other words, that when we feel an emotional state, our normal purposes and interests succumb to an influence beyond our control. The priority of emotions over will is important for our survival because it allows our plans to be interrupted by the immediate pressures of reality.

The priority of emotions over the will is also something we commonly resent. No one particularly likes being under control. Emotions are like our parents in this regard, annoying and cumbersome, pushy and old-fashioned, but probably doing things for our own good. This becomes all the more cloying when our emotions go on and on, signaling some vague threat or malaise, making us sad or afraid or filled with dread, and yet suggesting nothing obvious for us to do to discharge the feeling and go on with our lives. Like pain that has signaled a problem and gotten us to seek treatment, and then lingers without further usefulness, emotion can seem superfluous and cruel.

This, then, is what can occasion attempts at mood control. Typically, we don't try to suppress positive moods. Although we may occasionally have trouble with too much frivolity in serious circumstances, and so will attempt to rein in our snickering, it is the intrusion of negative emotion we most detest. A negative emotion or mood arises to signal to us that something is wrong, and either because we can't or won't fix that something, the emotion outstays its initial usefulness. It keeps interrupting, time and again frustrating our other motives and purposes. It is not surprising, when this happens, that the elimination of the mood may itself become our purpose.

Automatic Thought Cycles. What are we up against? One way of describing emotion is to say it is largely an automatic function, and that this is why it is so hard to control. This inevitable, automatic quality of a mood state is captured well in a simple image of the mind that is currently popular among some psychologists—the mind as a network of related ideas.[115] In this model, thoughts are linked in a mental network to the other thoughts that we associate with them, and thoughts are related to moods in this very way. For example, the mood of sadness may lead to remembering the day years ago when the beloved family dog was killed. By the same token, remembering that incident when one is in a normal mood could bring on the mood of sadness. An automatic network model of thinking predicts quite well why it is we typically think on themes in this way, finding that our moods are tied to certain realms of ideas.

There is experimental evidence for this sort of mental network. In some studies, for instance, it is found that if people are exposed to a word list when they are in a particular mood, they are later more likely to recall those words accurately when they are in the same mood. Likewise, happy readers are more likely to recall characteristics of the happy person in a story than are sad readers, and vice versa.[116] The intertwined influence of our moods and our thinking is sufficient for theorists who are attempting to understand severe mood problems such as clinical depression to rely on the same idea. They hold that depressed people arrive at their poor outlooks, and maintain such moods, by virtue of automatic thinking of negative thoughts.[117] What all this means is that negative thoughts cause bad moods, bad moods in turn cause negative thoughts, and the two thus can cycle back and forth to keep us in a sorry mental state for a long while.

The depressed person will spend a lot of time wallowing in the feeling. It is not easy to attempt to get out of this prison of thought, and sometimes the despair seems appropriate. Dostoevsky explained the magnetism of this emotion, and its origins in our cognitive activity, in *Notes from Underground:*

> And secretly, in my heart, I would gnaw and nibble and probe and suck away at myself until the bitter taste turned into a kind of shameful, devilish sweetness and, finally, downright definite pleasure . . . the pleasure came precisely from being too clearly aware of your own degradation; from the feeling of having gone to the uttermost limits; that it was vile, but it could not have been otherwise; that you could not escape, you could never make yourself into a different person; that even if enough faith and time remained for you to make yourself into something different, you probably wouldn't want to change yourself; and even if you did want to, you wouldn't do anything because, after all, perhaps it wasn't worth while to change. But finally, and chiefly, all this proceeded from the normal basic laws of intellectual activity and the inertia directly resulting from these laws, and consequently not only wouldn't you change yourself, you wouldn't even do anything at all.[118]

If this is how moods and thoughts cooperate, then mood change is bound to be very slow. We might be deeply depressed, for example, and be thinking about drowning. From this point, we might automatically remember a distant relative who drowned. Although this thought is almost as dreadful as the idea of our own drowning, it is not quite so bad—maybe we hadn't met that relative anyway. So, our next mood is just a tiny bit better than the previous one. After this, we may move to another thought that is ever-so-slightly better, and so on, so that over a long while we could, in small automatic steps, move out of the deep negative state in which we began. There could be reversals in this "random walk" through our thoughts, leading us again toward depression. Getting into a better mood could take days, weeks, or even months, depending on the severity of our initial depressed mood, and indeed such slow recoveries seem to be the rule. But people do seem to come back from even severe depression automatically, over time.[119]

It is only natural to want to speed this up. To do this, we must find some way to sidestep the automatic perpetuation of moods by thoughts, and thoughts by moods, that keeps our moods the same. Controlling our thinking is a good possibility. If we can concentrate on good things and suppress bad ones, we are going to be inclined to improve our moods in the bargain. It is interesting to note that this approach conflicts with the supposition that all mental change is best described in terms of automatic networks of thought linkages. Taking the helm and attempting to change thought patterns is a controlled thought strategy, one that could relocate your attention by jumps to very different areas of thought than might be found through automatic links alone. Any change that is attributable to such efforts can best be understood as occurring outside the usual automatic mental engines.

The professional way to control our emotions, of course, is to seek out a psychotherapist, someone who knows the ropes on thought control. Those who practice a form of *cognitive therapy* will usually be more than happy to recommend strategies for thought control.[120] The cognitive strategies that therapists will apply are usually indirect ones. Rather than calling for direct suppression ("Stop those bad thoughts") or concentration ("Start some good ones"), the therapist may suggest cognitive restructuring or problem solving.[121] Cognitive restructuring is an approach in which the person is encouraged to think differently about the mood-producing situation; say, over time one is led to view a divorce as the chance for a new life rather than the tragic end of an old one. Problem solving, in turn, is an approach in which the person is encouraged to think of a way to change the mood-producing situation; say, one might be prompted to overcome the divorce by going out and seeking new friends and contacts, buying a pet, or otherwise changing one's life situation to promote a new mood.

These techniques contrast with a direct approach, the attempt simply to avoid those negative thoughts that induce a bad mood, and to substitute instead positive thoughts that might yield a better mood. The direct approach has its adherents, too, as psychologists have often recommended just this way of climbing out of the blues.[122] Acting coaches, too, recommend mood control via the control of thinking as a way of making stage portrayals more genuine.[123] We should be cautious here, though. We have seen that the attempt to avoid an unwanted thought can be perplexing, and it is important to realize that direct control might backfire if it is not handled well. Direct mental control, however, is what this book is about, and it is crucial for us to examine just how it works in this case.

One more clue we have that mental control could be useful in controlling bad moods comes from clinical research. Studies of people who are deeply depressed indicate that they often suffer, too, from obsessional thinking, the inability to avoid recurrent unwanted thoughts. What is remarkable about this is that usually obsession precedes depression rather than the other way around.[124] It could be that an initial inability to control thoughts serves as an Achilles' heel, a weakness that allows people to slip into deeper and deeper negative moods, and eventually into severe depression. With this in mind, it becomes important to discern whether negative moods are controllable through thought suppression.

Eliminating the Negative.   People have been asked to suppress negative thoughts in laboratory experiments.[125] Participants for these studies were screened in advance to determine their mood state. Some were selected because they reported their moods to be normal, whereas others were selected for the study because they reported feeling depressed. The depressed participants were not so deeply depressed that they required medication or psychotherapy, but they reported thoughts and behaviors on a standard measure, the Beck Depression Inventory, that indicated they were at least moderately depressed.[126]

Each participant was furnished with either a very positive thought or a very negative one in the form of a story. One of the negative stories used in the study, for example, was as follows:

You have an important interview for a job. This job appears to be ideal in almost all respects. If you are able to get the job you will be receiving a terrific salary and benefits. In addition, you will be doing exactly the kind of work you most enjoy. Naturally, you are excited and find it difficult to fall asleep the night before the interview which is scheduled for 9:00 AM. Finally, you doze off at about 3:00 in the morning.

When you next open your eyes you slowly turn over in bed and glance at the clock. It's 8:30 AM! You forgot to set the alarm and now the interview is in 30 minutes! After hurriedly dressing you race to the car and speed off to your appointment. While driving you are aware that you are speeding but decide it's the only way you can get to the appointment on time. You look toward the upcoming intersection and see the light turn yellow. Although you are still a considerable distance from the intersection, you accelerate. As you approach the intersection you see the light turn red and you see a car beginning to cross. You hit the brakes but it's too late. You slam into the side of the car to the sound of screeching tires and smashing glass. The next thing you are aware of is a group of people standing over you. One of them tells you not to move, that help is on the way. As you turn your gaze away you see the driver of the other car with a small infant in her arms. You hear her cry out, "She's dead! She's dead! My baby is dead!"

This is a stark thought, one that bothers me even as I retype it now, and as you might imagine, participants in the study found it saddening indeed. A typical positive story used for this study, in contrast, led the reader to imagine being the hero in a happy incident, the finding of a lost child.[127]

Immediately after reading a story, each participant was asked to write down everything he or she was thinking, and to continue to do this for nine minutes. The experimenter signaled for the participant to begin writing on a new page every three minutes, so the course of the participant's thoughts over this interval could be studied later on. For some of the participants, this was the only instruction. Others were given an additional instruction to suppress the thought: They were asked to try not to think about the story they had just read, to make an effort to keep the story out of their minds. The written reports were then analyzed to see how many times each participant had mentioned the story over the nine-minute session.

The graph in Figure 5 shows how many times people mentioned the negative story. The most obvious result is that thinking about the story decreases across the three time intervals for most everyone. The normal (nondepressed) participants in the study (the dotted lines) showed this effect very clearly; they mentioned the story less and less over time. The depressed individuals (the solid lines), on the other hand, showed a decline in such mentions only if they were merely writing what was on their minds, and not trying to suppress the thought. Those who

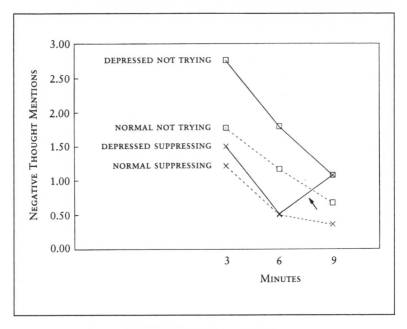

Figure 5. DEPRESSED VS. NORMAL PEOPLE
SUPPRESSING A NEGATIVE THOUGHT
OR NOT TRYING TO SUPPRESS

were instructed to suppress the thought did so effectively at first, and then—as shown at the arrow—they began to think about it again at the end. In fact, their level of mentioning was exactly the same at the end as the level of those depressed participants who had not even tried to suppress the thought.[128]

What is happening here? The depressed people in this experiment appear to suffer from an inability to suppress a negative thought. Nondepressed people do this rather well. And, although it is not shown in this graph, it was found that depressed people were quite good at suppressing a positive thought. (Small solace for those of us in bad moods—that we seem to be highly skilled at ridding our minds of pleasantries.) What the depressed person seems uniquely incapable of doing is eliminating an unpleasant thought from mind at will. The attempt produces a resurgence of negative thinking that occurs *even while thought suppression is still being attempted.* This is unlike the rebound effect found when normal people are asked not to think about white bears. That occurs *after* they have been released from the suppression and are invited to think about the white bear. These results show that depressives suffer a marked resurgence of an unwanted negative thought that begins even as they attempt to stop the thought.

There are several possible explanations for this. The most obvious one is that the automatic thought processes underlying depression are simply stronger than any attempts to control one's thinking. A more subtle way of looking at this, however, is probably closer to the truth. Perhaps when the depressed person attempts to suppress, he or she uses a poor self-distraction strategy. After all, we have learned that self-distraction is a key process in suppression, and this is an important place to look for faulty tactics in this case. If, for instance, the depressed person typically engages in self-distraction by choosing negative distracters, we would expect a pattern of suppression failure much like this one.

Perhaps in depression we get ourselves into a muddle by trying to push away from one negative thought by focusing on another. We try not to think about the possibility of getting fired at work, for example, by reflecting instead—of all things—on what it would be like if a loved one were involved in a hunting accident. These thoughts are quite distant from one another on some dimensions, but they share a very negative emotional tone. So, as compared to a distracter with a more positive or even neutral feeling, the negative distracter is more likely to induce a chain of thought that quickly comes round to remind us of the original unwanted thought. Our automatic association mechanisms can get more easily from the hunting accident back to getting fired than they could from, say, the thought of a trip to the Bahamas.

The written reports that were made by the depressed and nondepressed participants in the study were examined for evi-

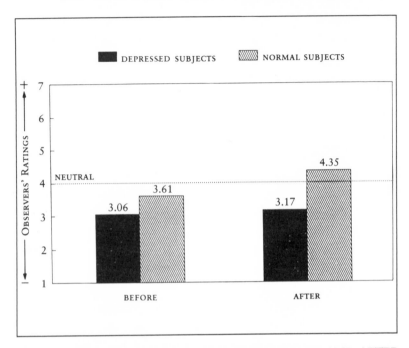

Figure 6. HOW POSITIVE ARE THOUGHTS BEFORE AND AFTER
MENTIONS OF UNWANTED NEGATIVE THOUGHT?

dence of such a strategy difference. What was the emotional
tone of the thoughts people wrote during the experiment? The
important comparison was between those thoughts people had
just before an intrusion of the thought they were instructed to
suppress, and those they had *just after* such intrusions. The ones
just before are probably the things that reminded them of the
unwanted thought, whereas the ones just after are probably
things they were thinking in order to distract themselves from
that thought. Figure 6 shows the emotional tone of those
thoughts for depressed and nondepressed participants as they
attempted to suppress a negative thought.

The findings demonstrate that depression does produce a
faulty strategy for self-distraction. You will notice at the left
side of this graph that both depressed and normal participants

were reminded of the unwanted negative thought by similarly negative ideas. Both groups wrote sad things just before the sad story returned to mind. Their automatic reminding mechanisms, in other words, were working just the same—and quite well. The normal individuals, then, attempted to counter the intrusion of the unwanted negative thought by moving to a positive thought after the intrusion. As shown on the right side of the graph, the normals think something positive after they've finished with the negative unwanted thought. This sets them on course away from the negative side of their minds, and makes it less likely that they will drift back to the unwanted negative thought. The depressives seem to have missed this point entirely. They thought about something negative after the intrusion, their meager self-distraction attempt leaving them still perilously close to the negative thought that they were trying to suppress.

Now remember: We are looking here at just the people who were given an explicit instruction to suppress a negative thought. They were in a psychology experiment and they knew it. They probably were feeling some pressure to perform, to do the right thing. But the depressed people in this experiment chose a clearly self-defeating strategy nonetheless. They tried to pull themselves away from the negative thought by reflecting on other negative thoughts, and this doomed their attempts at suppression. It is no wonder they experienced a resurgence of the unwanted negative thought before the experiment was over.

Could depressed people be so blind that they don't even realize a positive thought would be the best to distract them from the negative? A second study was conducted in this series to see whether the problem was indeed this severe. When both normal and depressed people were asked what they *should* do, there was little difference. Like nondepressed people, those who felt depressed were perfectly capable of volunteering the right strategy when they were asked point blank what would be most effective. What, then, is getting in the way of the depressed individual?

Accentuating the Positive. The automatic thought network could be responsible for the self-defeating strategy that depressed people use. It could be that they simply pick a self-distracter from thoughts that come to consciousness quickly and easily. And maybe in depression, positive thoughts usually lose the race to negative thoughts. The depressed person may want to find a positive self-distracter, but nothing along this line comes to mind soon enough to do the job. One tactic that might work, then, would be to provide possible distracters to depressed people. If there were some nice, shiny positive thoughts out there to reflect on, perhaps they could enact the proper strategy and suppress negative ideas more successfully.

This opportunity was given to a number of depressed and nondepressed people in a third experiment. In this study, participants were asked to suppress a negative thought presented in a story. Immediately after they read the story, they were instructed to begin writing about any of nine topics that were presented. The topics ranged from positive ("falling in love") to neutral ("walking down stairs") to negative ("getting sick"). Keep in mind that now, potential positive distracters are provided and the trouble of having to think them up should no longer get in the way. Depressed people should be able to pick them and use them—*if* they are aware of the effective self-distraction strategy.

Depressed people in this study did tend to choose the right distracters. They chose more positive than negative things to think about as they were trying to get away from the negative unwanted thought. But they still didn't do this nearly as well as nondepressed people. As you can see in Figure 7, the tendency to choose positive over neutral and negative distraction topics is very strong in normal people. They seem to want very much to think of something good to get away from something bad. But this inclination is much weaker in depressed people. There is still the choice of positive over negative, but it is only a slight preference rather than a resounding one.

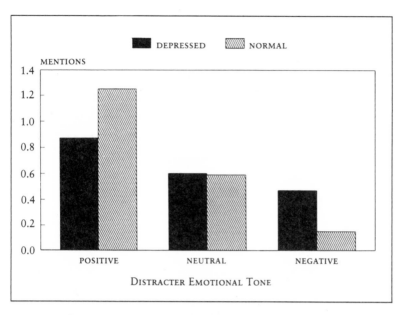

Figure 7. USE OF AVAILABLE DISTRACTERS
FOR SUPPRESSING NEGATIVE THOUGHT

In light of this, it seems there is a way out of depression. It is a dark, winding path, one that not everyone can travel. The light at the end of the tunnel is this: In the depths of a depressed mood, people still know enough to show a preference, albeit a feeble one, for positive thoughts to use as self-distracters. This means that if such thoughts can be made available to them, they may begin to use them in the attempt to control their moods. Without such externally provided positive ideas, of course, there is not as much hope. The automatic thought network will just keep pushing negative thoughts forward whenever a distracter is sought, and in this way undermine what could become an effective technique for mood control. It takes *available* positive distracters to aid in any bid to improve one's mood.

We spoke in an earlier chapter of the remote control of thinking, the manipulation of external stimuli in the campaign to control our minds. It may well be that this is the best advice we have to offer about depression as well. The battle of mood may be won only when we can fight the automatic negative thoughts within by enlisting positive thoughts from outside. If we hang around happy people, sit in pleasant places, and look at good things, we will have a constant array of positive thoughts to use as self-distracters. We may not always use them, and our poor mood may make us stand out as party-poopers amidst all this joy. But with these circumstances, we make available to ourselves the good thoughts that we otherwise cannot seem to dredge from the depths of our mind. We may begin to find some success when we apply the self-distraction strategy. It appears that direct mental control of mood is most effective when it is supplanted by indirect methods—changes in one's situation that allow attention to focus on helpful distracters.

The only other alternative is to wait. As we have learned, it is probably the case that our sluggish and conservative mental network will eventually walk us away from our poor mood. This automatic process could take a long time. If we want to do it faster, to take control, then external reminders of good things will be among the most useful aids we can have. It would be nice if we could agree completely with Rodgers and Hammerstein that remembering our favorite things will make us feel better. Remembering our favorite things is not so simple, though, when we are deep in sadness. We must surround ourselves with these things, revel and bask in them, celebrate them and search for them, and even when they are all around keep reaching for more.

There is a lesson in this idea for the control of all moods, not just depression. Let us take the example of test anxiety, a feeling that is at least a step or two away from the depressed moods we have considered thus far. The student who is afraid of performing poorly on a test will usually have some trouble with thoughts that automatically reinstate the anxious mood: "I will fail the test," "My mind will blank completely when I start," "The rest of the students will all finish first," and perhaps even

"I'll be so nervous I'll be sick." These thoughts produce the mood and are produced by it. As the test starts, the thoughts and the mood escalate wildly, each in response to the other. In the midst of this emotional turbulence there is no way out.

What is needed here is much the same strategy we just described for controlling depression. The control of problems such as test anxiety can be aided by increasing the availability of proper distracters. The best possible distracters from the fears of failure during a test, of course, are thoughts of great success and triumph during the test. These distracters are entirely opposite the thoughts that you would like to suppress, and their availability would help a lot just when that automatic storm of failure-related thoughts begins to form. Just as the class is starting and the tests are being distributed, however, thoughts of success are nowhere to be found. They might as well be encased in concrete somewhere for all the difficulty you have in bringing them to mind.

The way to have appropriate distracters available is to prepare them in advance. Making a list of success thoughts could be relatively easy the night before, or perhaps a few weeks before, and with this in hand one might be better prepared to engage properly in self-distraction. Research has shown that the early preparation of potential positive thoughts in situations like this can be very helpful.[129] A handy list of self-distracters could be useful for many mood-producing situations—when we can predict them in advance. If we know a test is coming up, a breakup with a lover is inevitable, an angry confrontation with a coworker is going to happen soon, or the like, we may be able to help ourselves avoid some of the unpleasant emotional cost of these things. Armed in advance with cognitive ammunition—thoughts that are opposite those associated with the mood, and that we therefore will find useful in distracting ourselves—we may be more successful in fighting unwanted emotions.

The Automatic Shield. In all of our concern with controlling negative moods, we have neglected to this point to consider what positive moods are like. Knowing what they are like may help us to hold on to them while we have them, so it is worthwhile to consider the opposite of a bad mood. Although good moods may feel to us like a night-and-day change from the bad ones, there is reason to believe that they operate on very similar principles. Good moods, too, seem to exist in an automatic interplay with associated thoughts. Positive thoughts give rise to good moods, and good moods to positive thoughts, in a continuous process that makes positive moods fairly stable as well.[130]

Thinking bad thoughts may not change our good mood, or even a neutral one. The mood serves as an automatic shield that protects us from negative thoughts. "Wonderful," you say to yourself, "at least the appalling sluggishness and uncontrollability of our minds is good for *some*thing." And you are very right. We are fortunate indeed that our moods are not jerked around by every nasty thought that comes by, or even by every whim we have about what mood we should be feeling. The automatic shield of a positive mood guarantees that it will take a very absorbing thought—something *really* bad, or a succession of at least fairly bad ones—to break through and get us concentrating on the negative.

The emotional protection that is offered by our network of positive thoughts is often called a psychological "defense." Freud and others since have spoken frequently of the idea that people may fend off threatening or unflattering information by virtue of some mental mechanism of this kind. Clear defensive purposes seem to be involved, for instance, in the fact that people typically take credit for their successes but blame their failures on bad luck or contrary circumstances.[131] People usually claim that they are happy, that things are looking up in the future, that nothing is wrong with them, that they will get a job if they don't have one, and that their children will be more gifted than normal. They also believe that bad things such as accidents, illness, unemployment, or becoming the victim of a crime are less likely to happen to them than to others.[132] This glow of optimism outshines many of the dark shadows that can loom over our lives.

The automatic shield does not come without drawbacks, however. In the rush to continue thinking positive thoughts in the face of incoming negative information, we may automatically shield ourselves from reality. It has been found, for instance, that depressed people are better able to judge when something they are doing is useless. Nondepressed individuals continue to believe that they are having some influence even when their activities have no real impact on what is happening around them.[133] It may well be that the automatic shield we carry leads us frequently to overestimate our successes. We live in a universe of illusion, perceiving ourselves and our world to be better than they are.

What is the harm of this? Occasionally, the automatic shield will lead us to get out on a limb and chop it off. We may overestimate how well we are doing on a date, for example, and propose marriage before our partner has fully committed our name to memory. We may arrange business deals on the assumption that everything has always gone well, is going well, and will go well—and send all our money down the well. Without such confidence, we might never do anything risky at all. But with such confidence, we are bound always to bite off a bit more than we can chew.[134] The very uncontrollability of our positive outlook on life makes us attempt to control our worlds just a shade more than we can.

All these futile attempts, broken dreams, and unrealistic desires can make us seem crazy at times. Although we are perfectly "normal," we have a bit more of a "manic," hyperactive glint in our eye than does someone who is truly depressed. Normalcy, in a way, is its own kind of problem, an illusory state that seems precarious when we view it from a depressed mood. But the automatic shield is not particularly precarious at all. It is just as stubborn and unmovable, in its own way, as the cage of negative thoughts we languish in when we are depressed. These automatically activated mental states are largely responsible for what we feel.

Mood control is possible because we can control our thoughts. But the work of controlling moods is slow. We must be calculating at times, arranging our situations and preparing ourselves, so we can supply our minds with the mood-related thoughts that automatic processes fail to supply. But given the availability of such distracters, we can have some success in suppressing the thoughts that promote our most unwanted moods. Luckily, the leisurely pace of our mood changes usually works for us rather than against us. Our normal moods and positive thoughts intertwine to form a network that catches and rejects all but the most insistent annoyances. Their shield prevents us from overreacting to the life events that might otherwise shake our emotional life every moment.

EIGHT

Exciting Thoughts

If the mind, which rules the body, ever forgets itself so far as to trample upon its slave, the slave is never generous enough to forget the injury; but will rise and smite its oppressor.

—Henry Wadsworth Longfellow, *Hyperion*

Imagine you are in the presence of a strikingly attractive person, someone you would love to cuddle forever. You are excited, basking in the glow of the person's nearness, but it is not appropriate to say or do anything about it. You are married, perhaps, or the person is your boss's spouse, or yet something else stands in the way. So, you throttle your desires and try to ignore the romance. You may even succeed at this for a while, to the point that you can actually carry on a conversation about the weather. But your body can't forget. You are flushed, maybe a bit jumpy, and your hands keep quivering. If you're like me, at this point you will probably spill something or step in the dog dish. Your mind is unable to keep control and your body is running the show.

Each human mind is carried around, serviced, and ultimately constrained by an elegant sack of meat, a body. So far in this book, we have managed to stay in the world of the mental and ignore this fact almost entirely. We have singled out mental control processes and considered their intricate workings without once appreciating the physical prop on which they stand. But this neglect must stop. The body will announce itself. It gets short of breath, its heart races, it sweats, it tingles, it gets numb, it shakes and shivers, it aches, its stomach turns, it has orgasms, it gets sick, and it reports its presence in a hundred other ways. Mental operations are accompanied by bodily states, good or bad, and the body cannot be overlooked.

This chapter is about how mind and body influence each other in the struggle for mental control. At the heart of this complex issue are the anxiety and nervousness that often accompany unwanted thoughts. When we have unwanted thoughts that cause such reactions, we usually say we are "worried" or "anxious"—and we try to wish the thoughts away. After all, these thoughts seem to be the source of unwanted symptoms such as muscle tension or trembling, cold hands, shortness of breath, or yet others. But our attempts to escape the thoughts that cause these reactions can eventually aggravate and perhaps even prolong the very symptoms we wish to avoid. The struggle to control the mind may lead us to lose control of the body.

Up on the Roof.   My office is in a four-story building, and there is a stairway to the roof just down the hall. I've been on the roof before, as it is a good vantage point for fireworks displays on the Fourth of July. The roof has no railing at the edge, and a nagging fear of heights keeps me well back from the rim whenever I'm up there. Once when I was with a group of friends on a holiday evening, a slightly inebriated member of our party went over and sat on the edge, legs dangling and wiggling, to watch the display. There is gravel on the roof, and it is slippery. I called him back, as did others, but he sat there defiantly. I saw not a single firework that night. Instead I looked in every other direction to avoid glancing at someone who, I felt, was a dead man. All I need to do even now to get a slight case of nerves is have this image come to mind.

Occasionally, it does. One afternoon, for some reason I am reminded of that night on the roof—and I get a shiver. But curiously, the same shiver is not forthcoming when I sit down and concentrate on the thought for a while. Sure, the internal stir is still noticeable. But it takes some time turning the thought over in my mind to find a new aspect of it that is exciting before I get a shiver again. I happen to recall, for instance, a remark someone made about going up to play Frisbee on that railingless roof and I get a bodily reaction again. But if I dwell on it a while longer, even this seems to lose its bothersome quality and I need to invent something else to bring back that shiver. Eventually, I put the whole thing out of mind and get back to work.

Days, weeks go by. And then, again, out of the blue I get hit with that crazy thought of squirming on the gravelly edge. I get a high-voltage shiver, one that seems every bit as alarming as the original. It seems my bodily reaction to this exciting thought is unusually severe *when I have successfully suppressed the thought and it suddenly intrudes on my consciousness.* It doesn't seem quite so bad when I purposefully focus on the thought. This observation is at the heart of an important realization about the unwanted thoughts that upset our bodies. In essence, such thoughts are empowered by our attempts to suppress them. The bodily reactions we experience when we have exciting or disturbing thoughts may be strengthened and perpetuated by our attempts to suppress the thoughts.

Suppression in a short while can settle us down. It puts the exciting thoughts out of our conscious awareness, and so stops the normal tendency of such thoughts to charge us with anxiousness. But when the suppression is complete, we then have made ourselves into sitting ducks, oblivious to the very thoughts that will surely disturb us if we are reminded of them by any random ideas or cues. In this position, it is no wonder that we are unpleasantly surprised when the unwanted thought returns. We experience a special surge of alarm, an *intrusion reaction,* when the thought comes back to mind. This happens after every attempt at suppression, in a way fueling the fires of our tension each time we hope to throw water on the flames.

Normally, people don't surprise themselves. No matter how loud you yell "boo" at yourself, no matter how long you wait in a dark corner before you spring out waving your arms, it doesn't work. Like tickling yourself or telling yourself a joke, surprising yourself is an odd occurrence, the result of an unusual *division* within yourself. In order to make a true self-surprise, you must become estranged from part of yourself so that a "surpriser" part can be psychologically separate from a "surprisee." This seems very odd, and it is easy to write off such dissociation of oneself into parts as a weird phenomenon, perhaps even something like "multiple personality" or some other kind of rare disorder.[135] There is at least one common example, however, that suggests we can indeed surprise ourselves in much this way without being abnormal at all.

Consider what happens when you have a memory on the "tip of your tongue." You try repeatedly to recall a movie title, a song lyric, someone's name, or the like—but it just isn't coming. You finally set the whole problem aside, even though you know that you should be able to reproduce it. Later that day, though, or perhaps the next, it hits you like a truck. You jump up and yelp "Escape from the Planet of the Mules"—or whatever it was. You have retrieved a memory that you were on the lookout for, and when it hit, you clearly experienced a surprise. It is as though some sort of unconscious search mechanism had been set ticking in the background of your mind the whole time, waiting and watching for a cue that would set off the retrieval of the desired memory. When the item was finally retrieved, you surprised yourself.[136]

This is the same basic event that happens when a previously suppressed thought returns to mind. Instead of an unconscious search mechanism that is looking in the background for an unretrieved memory, however, there is instead a mechanism that is searching for an occurrence of the suppressed thought. After all, part of successful suppression is remembering to avoid the thought, and there is thus good reason for part of the mind to be on the lookout in this way. This search mechanism is not one that we are thinking about consciously, of course, as that would constitute thinking the unwanted thought itself. But the search mechanism churning in the back of our minds keeps the unwanted thought highly accessible to consciousness, and makes it likely that we will be alert to the thought when it arrives. Like the air traffic controller who is continually watching for signs of a potential mid-air crash, and who therefore snaps to attention when any sign is found, the person tuned to find the return of a suppressed thought will surely notice it and react with alarm to its intrusion.

This, then, is the main focus of this chapter: how our nervous reaction to disturbing unwanted thoughts is aggravated by the suppression of those thoughts. To understand in detail how this happens, we need to examine how the body reacts to exciting thoughts, how suppression initially acts to remove the bodily reaction, and how this intended effect comes to backfire and make the bodily reaction more violent than it would have been had we never tried to suppress the thought at all. We will consider each step in turn.

Exciting Thoughts and Arousal. How do thoughts make us nervous? In some cases, the connection between a thought and a bodily reaction seems obvious. When we have fears or desires, we have a good idea of what thought caused the bodily excitation.[137] In other cases, it is not so clear why we feel as we do. Freud popularized the notion of "anxiety" early in the history of psychology by pointing out that people could also have states of nervousness that were not traceable to particular thoughts.[138] He held that anxiety is noteworthy primarily because of this—its origin is a mystery to the person it inhabits. Contemporary psychological theory echoes this distinction between known and unknown sources of excitation.

In both cases, the excitation is the same. When people say they feel nervous or emotionally upset, for whatever reason, they will also commonly report one or more physical symptoms—upset stomach, tense muscles, racing or pounding heart, difficulty in breathing, cold hands or feet, sweating, quivering, sinking feelings in the stomach, tension headache, dryness of the mouth and throat, or weakness in the limbs.[139] These symptoms are traceable to a general pattern of activation in the body, a pattern associated with the secretion of adrenaline (epinephrine) by the adrenal glands. It is called the sympathetic activation of the autonomic nervous system,[140] and it usually accompanies our conscious perception that we are upset.[141] The occurrence of such excitement does not depend on our knowing *why* we are upset.

This pattern of activation is the one you may feel when you drink too much coffee. The same symptoms, and the feeling of nervousness, are part of emotions from joy and delight to rage, fear, and disgust. The flush of excitement that accompanies sexual arousal, for instance, features many of the same bodily symptoms as the experience of fear. There are some detectable differences: Sexual arousal has bodily indications in both males and females that distinguish it from the normal response to a looming thug. But the symptom differences among many emotional states tend to be far less noticeable, and measurable bodily distinctions between emotions are more the exception than the rule.[142]

Our bodies become excited in a general way, in short, no matter what is exciting our minds. We may be worried about falling, we may be angry at a store clerk who is taking too long to ring up our sale, or we may be quivering with pep at the thought of receiving a cheerleading award—and in each case have the same general syndrome of bodily change. This general change has been called *arousal*. According to a theory originated by Stanley Schachter and Jerome Singer, arousal is a central component in our experience of any emotion.[143] We do not feel emotions without it. Any noteworthy event leads us to become aroused, and our sensing of bodily excitement leads us to examine our circumstances to determine why we have this generalized feeling.

Often, the reason is obvious. We note we are standing in front of a critical audience with nothing on our minds to say, for example, and we immediately understand that the arousal is an instance of fear. But we may become aroused in a setting that does not allow us to understand as clearly what we are feeling, and then it may take us a while to discern why we are aroused: We may find ourselves nervous as we talk to a stranger at a party, for instance, and it may take us some time to decide whether the person is scaring us or attracting us. This theory holds, then, that our emotions are not as tightly bound to our experiences as we sometimes think they are. Rather, emotions arise from the interpretations we find for our arousal. Schachter and Singer showed, for instance, that a person given an injection of epinephrine will react with different emotions depending on how the arousal is interpreted. Someone not told that this injection will produce nervousness is inclined to become happy in the presence of a person who is clowning around, yet will become angry in the presence of a person who is showing signs of anger. If the injected person is alerted to the fact that the injection produces the symptoms of arousal, however, there is little tendency to adopt emotional states in this chameleonlike way. Knowing what has caused the arousal gives the person a ready label for the arousal, and a definition of the appropriate emotion is not sought in the current situation.[144]

Viewed in light of this theory, it seems useful to consider anxiety or nervousness a default label we use when we do not know how to explain our state of arousal. "I'm anxious" is the explanation we have to offer when we have searched our environment and our memories and cannot find anything that would appear to be a sufficient cause for our arousal. The state of being aroused and not knowing why can be unpleasant.[145] Arousal without a label tends to make one self-conscious as well, turned inward, and even self-critical in a search for understanding of one's state.[146] The question of why one is upset keeps appearing and reappearing, and there is a strong tendency to adopt any explanation that becomes available.

Despite the mild unpleasantness of the anxiety state, it can be preferable to a strong negative emotion. When the interpretation we have in mind for our arousal is extremely disturbing and unpleasant, we may prefer not to know why we are aroused. General anxiousness and nervousness are better than horrible fears of falling or flying or failing—or whatever is really at the root of our body-wracking fright. So, we suppress an exciting thought, removing the interpretation of our emotion from mind, in the attempt to dismantle the emotion. This means that we immediately turn the emotion from its meaningful form into mere anxiety, a residual sizzle that seems to dissipate over time. An emotion requires both arousal and a label, and when we suppress the label the arousal slips away.

Suppressing Exciting Thoughts. To a degree, this escape from the source of an emotional reaction must work. Otherwise, why would we even do it? Thought suppression seems in a relatively short time to bring some relief from the emotion and perhaps can undermine the anxiety by cutting off its source. Often, however, we fail to escape from the interpretation right away because of the difficulties we have with suppression. So, the thought goes away and returns again in a minute. And it is sent away again and it intrudes again. Each time, it creates arousal anew when it appears. And each time, we send it away in our rush to have the arousal recede again. Although we have attempted to suspend the animation of our bodies by the disturbing emotion, it may not take much to bring the emotion back to life.

Observations consistent with this idea have been made in laboratory experiments. In these studies, the bodily reactions people have to emotion-producing stimuli are recorded directly by equipment that monitors signs of arousal. Although the measures vary in different studies, one most common sign is *skin conductance level*. This is a measure of the degree to which the skin conducts an electrical current, and it increases when the skin reacts to bodily arousal by sweating. Another common sign of arousal is heart rate, and there are others as well. These measures are not all straightforward indications of sympathetic activation, as they do not all increase and decrease together or for the same reasons—but we can count on them as crude indices of a person's overall excitement.

In one study of this type, people were asked to try to avoid becoming upset by a grisly film of (faked) sawmill accidents. These individuals indeed reported that they had managed to suppress emotional arousal. As compared to people asked to become involved in the film and feel the emotion, they said they were cool and detached. But these same "detached" people showed remarkably greater bodily agitation as measured by their increased levels of skin conductance.[147] It is as though their minds were cleared of the emotion, but their bodies stayed upset. This finding indicates that trying to suppress an emotion *while the emotion-producing stimulus is present* yields the same or greater arousal than trying to experience the emotion.

Very similar findings have been reported in research that examined skin conductance in college men who were looking at pictures of nude women.[148] Some of the men were placed under "inhibitory" conditions. They were asked before they saw the pictures to think back to "memories that come to mind that involve your mother or your father." Although this was not checked in the study, it is probably the case that thinking about their parents did a good job of putting a damper on their inclination to think about and enjoy the pictures. The men who were called upon to suppress their responses in this way, however, showed higher levels of skin conductance when they saw the pictures than did the men who were free to react as usual.

As in the sawmill study, thought suppression does not appear to eliminate bodily agitation when a disturbing stimulus is present. In fact, it even appears that suppression in these circumstances may *produce* arousal. The next question of interest, then, is whether suppression also has this influence when we try to suppress an exciting thought in the absence of anything that will strongly remind us of that thought.

A test of this was arranged in our laboratory. College students were asked to spend a series of three-minute periods trying in turn to think, or not to think, about each of several different things.[149] Each student had sensors attached to his or her body to measure levels of some major indicators of arousal. The student was then invited to speak continuously into a tape recorder as he or she thought about, or suppressed thought about, each of the following: Mom, the dean of students (an endearing woman known to all students at the university), dancing, and sex. These topics were chosen to represent a range of different thoughts, one of which was clearly exciting.

Now, it was expected that thinking about sex would be arousing for these students, and it was. As shown in Figure 8, levels of skin conductance were elevated during "expression" of sex. The intriguing observation here is that *not* thinking about sex turned out to be equally arousing for them. Skin conductance was just as high while they suppressed thoughts of sex. They seem to have remained quite excited physically during suppression of sexual thoughts even though their minds were emptying of the thoughts. It is worth noting, though, that the students in this study experienced all the usual problems people have in trying to suppress a thought in the laboratory, and they still tended to mention the unwanted thoughts even near the end of each three-minute period. They certainly mentioned the thoughts far less during suppression than when they were asked to express the thoughts, though, so it is remarkable that their level of excitement was so high.

In a second study in this series, participants were given longer periods of time to perform their thinking tasks. They were given five-minute periods to think about, or stop thinking about, either sex (the exciting thought) or dancing (the less exciting thought). Under these conditions, it became clear that the heightened levels of skin conductance that appeared during suppression of

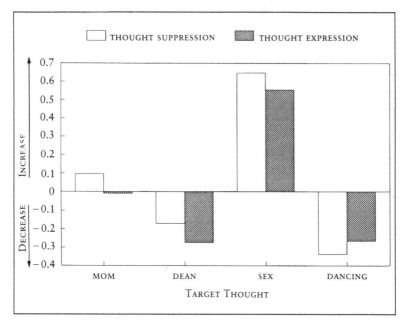

Figure 8. SKIN CONDUCTANCE LEVEL CHANGE

thoughts of sex were evident only in the *first two minutes*. This was the time during which participants had the most difficulty in eliminating the thought, and the bodily reaction appeared to dissipate as suppression continued past two minutes. This means that suppression *is* eventually successful in eliminating the strong bodily response to the exciting thought of sex.[150]

These experiments indicate thus far, then, that a person's level of skin conductance is heightened at first by an attempt to suppress an exciting thought, and that this level then goes down over the course of a few minutes. What then happens over a long period of time? A third study was undertaken in which participants were asked either to suppress or to think about an exciting topic (sex) or an unexciting topic (the weather) for thirty minutes at a stretch. And as you would expect, the number of times people mentioned the topic they were suppressing dropped over the time period—from several mentions in the first few minutes to almost none at all in the last few minutes. In comparison, mentions of the topic kept up at a moderate rate throughout the period among those individuals who were charged with thinking about their topic.

Our main interest was to learn how these mentions influenced each person's skin conductance level. For each subject, then, we examined the relationship between level of skin conductance and the tendency to mention the topic on a minute-by-minute basis over the half-hour session. And what we found was extraordinary: Among those asked to think about sex, there was no relationship; mentions of sex did not spur their arousal. Among people asked to think about the weather or not to think about the weather, there was no relationship; weather is not particularly exciting so, as we might expect, mentioning it did not produce arousal. Only among the individuals who were trying not to think of sex was there a connection. For them, mentioning sex in a particular minute produced an increase in skin conductance level during that minute.

This is direct evidence for the intrusion reaction. Apparently, when we are trying to think about something exciting (such as sex), each occurrence of the exciting thought does little to raise our bodily arousal. Although we may become more aroused overall when the topic is taken up, each new thought has little kick. Perhaps we are tuned to expect all the exciting thoughts that come to mind because we are actively steering our minds toward them—and so they lose their alarming quality. The individual thoughts of sex are not really individual occurrences at all, but part of an ongoing stream. And because the units of the stream are not separate, we do not react to them individually. However, when we are trying not to think the exciting thought, we find each new intrusion a source of arousal.

One way to understand this is to consider what happens when you stand in a moving stream of water. You might not notice the hundreds of buckets of water pouring over you because they all make up a single flow. However, if you were standing on a hot rock in the desert, you would notice a single bucket. Then, if you dried off and got hot again, you would surely notice the next bucket, too. And if you once again dried off, the next bucket would make for another fresh drenching. The state of mind we invite when we suppress an exciting thought prepares us, like the desert sun, to be newly surprised by each occurrence of the cold, wet thought.

This is not true, however, for thoughts that are not initially exciting. The results of the thirty-minute study showed that thoughts of weather were never linked to jumps in skin conductance level—when people were trying to think of weather, or trying not to think of weather.[151] There is something unique, then, about the special combination of exciting thought *plus* suppression that is not found with either exciting thoughts or suppression alone. The two together make each thought into an arousal-producing bullet, a disturbing intrusion that yields excitement each time it hits.

Deprived of Habituation.   One of the wonderful things that happens to us when we experience a negative emotion is that we get used to it. The most poignant sorrow, the most bone-chilling horror, the most revolting feeling of disgust, all tend to weaken somewhat the next time we experience them. People get used to jumping out of airplanes, they grow accustomed to getting hit in the face repeatedly in the boxing ring, they are benumbed by exposure to blood and horror movies. It seems to be a universal rule of psychology that people experience *habituation* to emotion-producing ideas and eventually find that little emotion is produced by them.

This "universal" rule does not apply to ideas we suppress. When we put an exciting idea out of mind, we seem to deprive ourselves of the privilege of getting used to it. Each new time it returns, we become excited again. The tendency to reject a disturbing thought the moment it jumps into view, then, is a counterproductive reaction. Although it produces immediate relief (well, at least after a minute or two of fussing with suppression), the long-term influence is to refresh the effectiveness of the exciting idea rather than to diminish it.

A study of people who have snake phobias is directly relevant to this.[152] Participants in this research were selected for their self-reported deep fear of snakes. Each participant was asked at first to review a stepwise sequence of different things one might do with regard to snakes—beginning with just thinking about one, and then moving up to looking at one from a distance, walking near it, picking it up, and so on. This was not pleasant at all for people who have snake phobias, and most would report wanting to stop at some point on the "ladder." When some of these people came to their personal stopping point, they were then encouraged to suppress their worry; they were told to visualize turning around and running from the snake.

Other participants arrived at their stopping points, only to be invited to think about it even more. They were given what clinical psychologists call "implosive therapy"—a big dose of snake thoughts. As it turned out, the heart rates of the people who were allowed to avoid the thought stayed high through several repeats of this sequence, one-hour sessions that took place over several days. The heart rates of the people who were asked to concentrate on the thought, in contrast, began *very* high but then declined over the course of these sessions. Because they faced the thought rather than suppressed it, their bodily reaction to the thought habituated. They got used to it.

Suppression typically deprives us of habituation. When I panicked on the roof that night and tried not to think of that clown out on the edge, I cut short the usual operation of my bodily reactions. I kept myself from getting used to the problem, and each time the frightening image returned later on I recoiled again and avoided any possible acclimatization. The quick and easy response I made to suppress the thought, in the long run, was what did me in. I now have a fairly well developed fear of heights in several situations, and I blame it on suppression. Lately, I've been trying to follow my own advice and actively seek out heights from time to time as a way of making myself get used to them. If at some time in the future you see a rather large gentleman plummeting toward the ground from a great height, you'll know that I finally habituated completely.

If there is any possibility that we might heal ourselves in such cases, it will probably begin with a commitment to try our best to get used to what makes us abnormally anxious or upset. It is important to do this gradually. For the person who has developed an extreme fear of getting AIDS, for instance, immediate contact with an AIDS victim could be far too disturbing to produce effective habituation. Such contact might yield a new round of thought suppression and so act to prevent the needed habituation. A more workable approach might begin with reading some pamphlets or even a book on AIDS. Talking about it with friends or a doctor might also be done without instigating suppression. Eventually, it might be possible to visit someone who treats AIDS victims, and even to meet and talk with victims themselves. If all of this could be done so gradually as not ever to start suppression, the extreme fear might well be overcome. Rather than suffering intrusion reactions each time the thought of AIDS came to mind, the person would have become used to the idea and have no special reaction at all.

Needless to say, this gradual approach is difficult to take because it requires a lot of thought about the very thought that is deeply unwanted just to program the steps of contact. This is why self-treatment for fears and phobias is not often as successful as visiting a therapist. Someone else who is not as bothered by the thoughts we fear may be able to help us become accustomed to them in a stepwise fashion. Although choosing not to suppress is an important first move in the enterprise of overcoming severe bodily reactions to thoughts, this choice may be one of the hardest ones there is because it must be made with each new occurrence of the unwanted thought. So it is useful to have help. It is also important to have alternative methods, and relaxation is a possible substitute when we cannot easily habituate.

Relaxation Time. Imagine for a moment that your chest hurts. It has been hurting for a few days, off and on, and you are worried. You look up chest pain in your home medical book, and it says terrifying things about heart problems and lung diseases. Sometimes when the pain is very noticeable, you get short of breath and can start feeling your heartbeat go faster—and these things are in the medical book, too. Is it the big one? One evening you actually get so upset you get shivers of panic and feel like your heart is stopping. But the moment passes, and the next morning you feel okay again and almost forget about it. A little twinge comes after lunch, and although you try to put it out of your mind all afternoon, it keeps on returning. So you avoid it some more.

People often proceed in exactly this way in the face of troubling symptoms that they fear may signal a major illness. The odd fact is that imagining possible severe consequences of an illness usually leads people to *delay* seeking medical care.[153] Trying not to think about the symptom is the standard reaction when severe negative consequences are imagined, and such suppression acts to allow people to put off getting aid. At some point, it will surely be necessary to see a physician and find out what is wrong. But if it turns out that the whole problem is anxiety or panic, the solution may be to work on the body directly. In this and a variety of other instances, habituation may be less important than simple relaxation.

Some people relax themselves chemically. They drink alcohol, and the repeated administration of this chemical produces a state of mindlessness and bodily sedation. In the short run, this often works in just the right way, as it tends to reduce the usual symptoms of anxiety and so can quell the urge to worry. In the long run, however, this strategy is likely to fail miserably. Alcoholism is not a particularly healthy road to mental control, as it brings a host of its own problems along that yield new and improved worries. There are better ways to relax.

The relaxation technique most widely used by clinical psychologists, and by many other practitioners, is the method of progressive relaxation developed by Edmund Jacobson.[154] I first came across a version of this in a Lamaze birthing method class my wife and I took when she was pregnant. The idea was to learn the technique so I could help her to relax during the anxious minutes between the contractions of childbirth. Sitting around on the floor in class with several other giggly expecting couples, we worked hard at it. My job was to help her focus attention on relaxing her body, one area at a time, by suggesting that she focus on each area and "let go" the muscle tension there. Her job was merely to follow the instructions (and of course, later, to have the baby).

Jacobson's method often begins with a basic exercise aimed at producing relaxation in one arm. A man who is attempting to relax in this way might be:

> . . . directed to "stiffen the arm without moving it, more so, still more, and still more! Then not quite so much, a little less, still less, and so on and on past the point where it seems perfectly relaxed, and even further!" He is requested to note that this is what will be meant by "going in the negative direction." *This is then taken as the type-form of progressive relaxation for all subsequent work.* It is necessary to warn (him) that one part of the illustration is not to be followed in the future: he should not as a rule contract before he relaxes, but should begin to relax at whatever stage he finds himself.[155]

The relaxation of that one arm, the "going in the negative direction," is then moved to the other arm, then to a shoulder, the other, and so on, in a pattern that covers all the major areas of body muscle from head to feet. If there are areas with special tenseness, the procedure may concentrate in that region. The basic plan, though, is to cover the whole body, allowing each muscle group to be felt and relaxed in a progressive pattern. (I should point out that many people have made the mistake Jacobson warned about—thinking that relaxation involves tensing and then relaxing each muscle group. Take special note that his method calls for you to start at normal and just relax—without any prior tensing. He used tensing only as an initial example to show what it feels like to relax from there.)

The method I learned in the Lamaze class had this same general idea. The plan was to concentrate on reducing the tension in various parts of the body, one by one, so that eventually the body as a whole would be relaxed. The class stressed the idea that this might be hard to do alone, and that the instructions of a "coach" would be helpful. Yet people use the technique alone with great success. Some methods of relaxation concentrate also on the importance of breathing and breath control; others include suggestions to clear one's mind, think of pleasant things, or attempt some form of meditation. Some methods involve playing audio or video tapes with a sequence of progressive relaxation instructions, often with music. All these methods use variations on this simple formula, and it works very well.

The problem with this technique is getting around to trying it. I'm quite sure that if I hadn't been trapped in a roomful of earnest people with my earnestly pregnant wife, I would never have learned the routine, let alone tried it. It seems somehow silly, a bit like pulling out the sleep mats during naptime in kindergarten. Spending fifteen minutes in a darkened room making my muscles relax is not my idea of a productive break, or at least not usually. It turns out now, though, that I find it very useful from time to time, and I'm glad I have this tool in my possession for when I might need it. When anxiety and worry start to escalate, this may be one of the few truly useful techniques we have to deal with them.

The use of relaxation is an indirect method of mental control. Rather than merely suppressing a worry, or distracting ourself mentally, we can *do* something, make a move that may help even though the worry is around. Moreover, we can use all the usual tricks of remote self-control to get going. We may set a relaxation time on our schedule every day, for example, or tell someone to hound us until we spend some time relaxing. We might get a partner to help us through the sequence, perhaps trading off with him or her every other time. We could buy a relaxation audiotape, or we could see a relaxation therapist to get us started.

There are yet other ways to get to the same place. Physical exercise, for example, is often cited as a potentially useful way of gaining relaxation, although there is not yet a great deal of research to indicate that it is a foolproof stress-reducer.[156] People also may use technology to aid in their relaxation attempts. Biofeedback devices—electronic signals that indicate bodily functioning in one or more areas—are potentially useful in this regard. These devices can be used to signal just how successfully one is relaxing a particular muscle system or reducing a specific indicator of arousal. There are a number of ways to get the body to follow the mind toward a relaxed, nonagitated state, and these are often worth exploring in the pursuit of peace.

Relaxation allows us the luxury of ignoring our body. Usually, its insistent signals tell us to worry about a particular thought. The thought that instigates arousal is something to be noticed and dealt with, and sometimes suppressed. But with relaxation, we may quell at least briefly those signals, and so avoid our strong impulse to suppress. In this way, relaxation may be an important aid to the process of habituation. We may get so relaxed that we can "take it" more easily when the exciting thought arises, and so wait longer before we feel the need to suppress the thought. In this waiting period, we get some time to get used to the thought, and so make it less likely that we will experience a strong reaction next time it appears.

The lesson of this chapter, to put it simply, is that body and mind must be controlled as a unit. Mental control alone will not work, as thought suppression may remove our worry only long enough to allow our body to be unpleasantly alarmed the next time we think of it. Habituation is what we really need, and suppression gets in the way of the body's natural tendency to accustom itself to disturbances. Relaxation is also helpful as a way to bring the body back to a normal state. But it must be realized that relaxation alone, too, is not enough. Relaxing the body will be insufficient if the mind is still upset. The same old worries may recur and they can instigate new bodily agitation in no time. Any attempt at controlling worry must be a concerted effort, a two-pronged attack at both bodily and mental disturbance. We must relax our body and soothe our mind, or the one that remains upset will soon stir up the other.

NINE

Synthetic Obsession

*Every impulse we strive to strangle broods in the mind,
and poisons us.*

—Oscar Wilde, *The Picture of Dorian Gray*

*I've been doing my best not to think about it, but by trying
so hard not to think about it, I can't stop thinking about it.*

—1986 Yankee shortstop Paul Zuvella during an 0-for-28 start

Sometimes an unwanted thought comes from an obvious source. You see a movie called *Blood Brunch*, for instance, and then you go home and get unpleasant flashbacks of bloody scenes later on. Anyone can tell what has produced your thoughts, although they probably won't show much mercy if you complain. After all, you brought this on yourself by going to the film. Many events that are beyond our control, however, can be tragically impressive to us in the same way. We experience something once—an accident, perhaps, or an act of cruelty—and then it is over. But soon we find we must live with mental replays of the experience. Such recurrent thoughts tend to portray the very events that gave rise to them, so their source is easy to identify.

Other unwanted thoughts, however, have more mysterious beginnings. How can we explain, for instance, recurrent thoughts of food, dirty hands, saying the wrong thing in public, dying, losing our keys, being mugged, or swerving the car into oncoming traffic? Nothing traumatic may have ever happened to us in these areas, but we may worry about them nonetheless. In these cases, it is unclear where the thought came from, and we may not even be able to say when it started to be unwanted. Yet such thoughts may have all the same qualities as a repeated thought that developed from a highly disturbing incident. These thoughts that sneak up on us, take over our minds, and keep intruding for what seems like no good reason are the topic of this chapter.

The basic idea is that people develop unwanted thoughts in one of two general ways. Either they experience some highly disturbing event, a trauma, and this leads to recurrent thoughts, or they experience a series of minor events that are much less noticeable, but that eventually build up to the production of the same sort of obsession. We will focus on traumatic obsessions first, and then turn our attention to the unwanted thoughts that appear with no clear beginning—synthetic obsessions. As we shall see, there is a good possibility that people suffer synthetic obsessions as a consequence of their unsuccessful attempts at mental control. Trying not to think of something may be largely responsible for making us continue to think it.

Traumatic Obsession. Many of the thoughts that people wish to suppress seem to be echoes, mental rehearsals of earlier events. This fact was recognized by Freud in his theory of neurosis, and has been observed in many different contexts.[157] The victim of rape, for example, is likely to have repeated thoughts of the event, including flashbacks and emotional surges that resemble a reliving of the event. These may take the form of nightmares about the assault, or more often occur simply as images during wakefulness. They can be accompanied by difficulty sleeping, physical symptoms, fears of being alone or with strangers, repeated washing, or persistent checking of locks or noises in what seems a desperate attempt to prevent an attack. Recurrent thoughts of revenge or violence to the rapist may occur as well.[158]

Trauma appears to etch a deep psychological scar in the

person. Like the rape victim, victims of all kinds often become obsessed with their traumas. The incest victim, for instance, may find that disturbing and painful thoughts of the traumatic events can last a lifetime.[159] The person who loses a spouse or child in a motor vehicle accident, too, will be likely to continue ruminating about the loss for years.[160] Witnessing a terrorist attack can have the same influence—the production of recurrent dreams and intrusive thoughts.[161] And of course, the experience of war can be traumatic to the extreme, affecting people's lives permanently and perhaps irrevocably, and leaving them forever to review the incidents they once endured.[162]

It is not entirely clear why traumas have this effect. Why should people be so deeply moved by traumatic events? The development of a full-blown obsession might take only a minute. The learning that occurs in this instant is so remarkably fast and thorough that it renders most other forms of life change or memory revision terribly slow and shallow by comparison. I remember as a child taking hours and hours of practice stretched out over weeks and sometimes months to learn one short piece on the piano—and now I've forgotten it completely. A trauma, in contrast, can make a person very different, very "wise" in a sense, and often in no time at all. The theories designed to explain this remarkable impact draw on one of three general ideas: massive memory reorganization, the need for complete emotional expression, or the posttraumatic operation of self-healing processes.

Traumatic obsessions might come from a massive emotional reorganization of memory. A trauma has a strong emotional component, and this emotion may serve to connect many different thoughts in our mind. When someone has died, for example, many things we think about are colored by our grief. It seems as though everything reminds us of the loss. This connectedness, then, may reinstate thoughts of the trauma whenever we are *not* thinking about it. This means that any negative ideas we encounter later on may lead us soon to think about the loss again. Our obsession with the loss may be the result of reorganizing our memories in terms of the trauma-induced emotion.[163]

The chronic repetition of thoughts after trauma could also be the result of an incomplete emotional reaction to the trauma. It could be that a given trauma requires a given amount of emotional expression: a death requires a certain cost in tears, perhaps, or physical abuse by one's spouse gives rise to a certain outcry. If such emotions are not expressed, they build up somehow and create an internal pressure for expression that results in the tendency to repeat thinking about the emotion-producing event. The notion of stored-up emotion was proposed by Freud, and has been reiterated by many contemporary theorists.[164] Such a "pressure-cooker" model of emotion suggests that the primary solution to traumatic obsession will be emotional expression.

The power of trauma to produce obsession might also be traced, however, to a very different sort of momentum. The reason we think about a trauma over and over may be that this thinking is good for us. The trauma may start in motion a natural process of self-healing or self-correction, in which the individual repeatedly reviews the trauma as a way of coming to terms with it and getting used to it—the habituation we have discussed before. The observation that parachutists keep exposing themselves to a highly disturbing stimulus—dropping to earth from a great height—and that they eventually get used to this, has prompted the idea that obsession or rumination may be a self-exposure technique. Perhaps the victim is trying to become inured to the idea of the trauma, and the repeated thought is a natural procedure for doing this.[165]

These theories of traumatic obsession cannot all be correct, of course, because they offer several contradictory ideas about how obsession arises and might be cured. Research is still going strong, and there is much to be learned before we can begin to decide which of these ideas may be a more useful approach to understanding and treating the problem. In the meantime, though, it is certainly worth noting that all the theories converge on one piece of advice for the traumatized: It may be *good* to think again and again about the trauma. Although this may seem like the most painful possible advice, and though it could be very wrong in some circumstances, there are some benefits to be derived from the obsession.

In terms of the "memory organization" theory, rethinking the trauma might help us by allowing us the time to see that the trauma is in fact *not* related to everything else in our lives. Of course, this realization must be added to our thinking, as it does not flow immediately from obsessing alone. But the rethinking of the trauma gives it a chance. In terms of the "emotional expression" theory, the advice is the same. The trauma will not be overcome until the emotion is fully expressed, and rethinking it is required. And the "self-healing" theory chimes in here, too. If obsession is a way of getting ourselves used to a trauma, then we should probably allow ourselves to do it. We will come back to this notion—that going with the obsession, experiencing it rather than suppressing it, might be a good idea. But first, we need to realize that not all obsessions can be traced to specific traumas.

Traumas are interesting, bizarre, gripping, and disturbing. We each have some of our own, and we can easily imagine the traumatic experiences of others. The notion that we relive traumas has a certain haunting romance to it, an aura of the tenderness and sensitivity of the human mind. Perhaps for this reason, the idea of a traumatic obsession is itself often overextended. Because it is so clear that people can get unwanted thoughts from traumas, there is a strong tendency for us to look for a trauma whenever someone has an unwanted thought. Freud started this with his notion that people exhibit neurotic symptoms—including obsessions—as the result of internal conflicts produced by childhood traumas.

It is true that relatively minor traumas can cause repeated

unwanted thoughts. In one study, for example, people saw some typical Hollywood horror film footage, and then were asked to report their subsequent thoughts and feelings. Many said they had intrusive thoughts about the film, ideas that interrupted their consciousness while they were thinking about something else.[166] You can probably remember a number of seemingly unimportant events that have reverberated in your mind in this way. In fact, you may not even believe that something has had an emotional impact on you until you later notice that it keeps coming back to your mind. These kinds of observations suggest we may search for some trauma, however small, at the beginning of almost every unwanted thought. Although this may not be the cause of the problem, we find it is the most likely culprit.

But what trauma is it that gives rise to repeated thoughts of cigarettes when someone is quitting smoking? And what trauma is it that makes someone keep thinking about the possibility that there will be no money left before the end of the month? Is there a trauma somewhere in the past of the husband who is obsessed about imagined infidelities by his wife? One might still look for traumas in these cases, and this is just what Freud tried to do. He insisted that traumas of one kind or another occurred so early in life that they were masked by childhood amnesia, the tendency we all have to forget most of the events of our early years.

Now, it is true that people don't remember much at all of their childhood years.[167] Major brain structures that allow us to knit our experiences together into retrievable memories seem not yet to be complete at this time, and there could well be early events that precipitate later obsessions.[168] The origins of unwanted thoughts in these murky beginnings of our minds are very difficult to trace, however, and it is not clear that these searches can ever reach satisfactory solutions. How will we know, even if we come across some childhood trauma, that it is indeed the one that has caused an obsessive thought in adulthood? Freud rendered this problem yet more complex by suggesting that traumas in one area in childhood (say, sexual ones) might produce obsessions in a very different area in adulthood (say, unwanted thoughts of dirtiness).

It is tempting in view of these complications to look for the beginnings of obsession where the light is better. Everything would be much simpler, after all, if we merely abandoned the insistence on traumatic origins in every case. Perhaps some proportion of our unwanted thoughts come not from traumas and instead have arisen from more mundane beginnings. A series of other events, all relatively nontraumatic, and thus uninteresting and easy to overlook, may have come together to produce these mysteriously repetitive thoughts. What could these little events be?

The best candidates are usually invisible to us. Whenever we find we have an unwanted thought, we tend to focus attention on the thought. We puzzle over what it means, how it is related to other thoughts, or simply over how to get rid of it. What we do not notice is the fact that we keep trying to reject the thought from our consciousness. Unwanted thoughts that occur too often and intrude on our minds may arise from our attempts at mental control gone overboard. Small initial attempts to control our thoughts could fail at first, leading us to escalate to more and more urgent suppression tactics. The need for suppression could grow, not because the thought was initially so intrusive, but rather because the suppression itself highlighted the thought and made it seem worth yet greater attempts at control. In short, we may develop disturbing obsessions with certain thoughts because, before they even began to obsess us, we tried to suppress them.

The Synthesis of Obsession. An obsession can grow from nothing but the desire to suppress a thought. We have seen that thought suppression often seems like the appropriate thing to do. When we try to gain self-control, we may suppress thoughts of the behavior or object we are avoiding. When we try to keep secrets, we may suppress thoughts of the idea that we are keeping from others. And when we desire to hold back an emotional expression, we may also attempt to suppress thoughts—in this case, thoughts that would normally make that emotion show itself. These wellsprings of suppression all can produce unwanted thoughts, each in its own way.

None of these sources of suppression seems at first to be strong enough or persistent enough to bother us very much. Imagine, for instance, the mental state of a devout Catholic adolescent girl who one day has a fantasy about the young priest at her parish. She keeps this little crush a secret, of course, and almost forgets about it completely. She is reminded of her thoughts later in church when he is around, and even though she gets a little shiver from looking into his watery blue eyes, she suppresses the thought at that time. So far, so good. In all likelihood, her attraction will turn out to be replaced by a different crush soon enough, and even this once-suppressed thought will escape the road to obsession.

But imagine how things might progress. Suppose that she nearly blurts out the fact of her whimsical attraction the next day at school, but then realizes just in time that the best friend she is telling is Catholic, too. What if it gets back to the priest, or to everyone at school? She decides that it is better to be quiet. But from this point on, the presence of her best friend reminds her to suppress the thought of the crush. The rest of the day she tries not to think about Father Blue Eyes. She goes home and, alone in her room, finds it is perfectly okay to think about him again. She starts to draw his picture in a notebook and ends up spending a whole evening thinking about her forbidden love. Her movement from a place that requires suppression—her friend's presence—to a place that allows expression—her room—gives rise to the first inkling of an obsession.

Remember that the rebound of unwanted white bear thoughts takes place under exactly such conditions. First, the person tries not to think of a white bear. Then, the person is allowed to do this. And in this period of license, there is the rebound, the tendency toward a special preoccupation with the formerly suppressed thought. It is very possible that this rebound could occur for many people in many circumstances, including for our lovelorn adolescent in her room, and this phenomenon could thus start the ball rolling. Still, this is probably not enough to create what we would classify as a Grade A Prime Obsession. Rather, it leads to just a bit more thinking about the unwanted idea than might be devoted to some other random idea.

The next step is the repetition of this sequence. Suppose that the girl is in her room, indulging her daydreams about the priest, when her friend drops in. The drawing of him must quickly be covered up, and all the wonderful visions of his company must now be suppressed. This is even more difficult than it was at school, and she keeps pushing back images of him as she tries to make conversation with her friend. The struggle to suppress a thought *during* a period of rebound from a previous suppression is especially difficult, and thus the suppression must go on longer and take more attention.

This could happen yet again, and perhaps over and over. She writes his name on her desk while daydreaming at school, for instance, and then must quickly scribble over it when her friend leans over to look. She gets so upset about it one day that she wants to tell her teacher, a nun, and get it off her chest. But she holds back at the last moment. She keeps getting caught in the rebound by new pressures to suppress, and each time it seems harder to do the suppression. The rebound is elevated each time as well. If this were to go on through enough repetitions, it would not be surprising to find that an extraordinary preoccupation had developed. She might pine away for months, perhaps even for years, waiting to be united somehow with her impossible love. Under our noses, an obsession was synthesized from what at first was merely a whim.

This process can be described as a *positive feedback* system, a cyclic process in which each occurrence of the cycle amplifies an initial signal.[169] The loud squawks that can come from a poorly adjusted PA system are the result of such positive feedback. When the microphone picks up some little sound, this passes to an amplifier that makes it louder, and then continues to the loudspeaker. But the microphone is still on, and it picks up the noise from the loudspeaker, sends it on to the amplifier where it is once again stepped up in volume and sent to the loudspeaker. Each loop of the noise increases its volume, and in an instant the room is filled with an obnoxious "BLOOOT." To fix it, one must turn down the amplifier or place the mike farther away from the speaker.

Suppression and expression of a thought escalate in response to each other in this fashion. The release of suppression leads to a rebound of expression, and this then requires a greater level of suppression to eliminate. The greater suppression, in turn, may yield a still greater rebound, and the cycle goes on and on—eventually to produce a thought that is alarmingly frequent and insistent, and can be suppressed only with great effort and concentration.

Many of the thoughts we try to suppress seem to become overly important to us through the operation of these *indulgence cycles*. An indulgence cycle is the move from suppression to expression that prepares the way for further suppression. Trying not to think about food works at first as a diet strategy, for example, and may even get us thin enough that we can allow ourselves once more to think about food. But in no time, a series of these cycles of indulgence can leave us totally obsessed and fat enough to scare the dog. Trying not to think about a dangerous behavior such as jumping in front of a bus, meanwhile, is also at first a wise thing to do. But if we then happen to let the thought out, only to suppress it once more, and so on in several cycles of indulgence, we may end up deeply worried that we will throw ourselves in front of the next bus we see.

This may seem odd indeed, and one wonders whether severe obsessions can really spring from such nuances. But repeated cycles can make small things into big ones, often much more quickly than we would guess. There is the story about a man who settled a bet by asking for a penny—to be doubled every day for a month. The money multiplied so rapidly in these daily cycles that it ended up being millions of dollars. The point here is that a relatively few occurrences of an indulgence cycle could yield the startling magnification of a small unwanted thought into a major obsession.

There are probably still other circumstances that must be right for an obsession to develop in this way. In the case of our Catholic schoolgirl, for instance, an obsession might best be promoted if she had little else to occupy her mind—the schoolwork was easy, for example, or she was uninterested in it. Feeling isolated and different from others might help, too, as it would make her think that her initial thoughts were somehow so weird or different that no one else could possibly consider them to be normal. Even the timing of suppression and expression might be critical, and certain other sequences of events might have left her with no obsession at all. It is probably not the case that every suppressed thought yields an obsession over time, but rather that only a few are selected by a particularly fertile circumstance to become deeply unwanted thoughts.

Our bodies are involved in all this as well. As noted previously, the suppression of anxiety-producing worries may often leave us ready to experience a severe intrusion reaction when the worries return. In suppressing the thought, we stop ourselves from getting used to it and instead make ourselves highly sensitive to its next occurrence. So, each time it happens we get unusually upset. Such processes could act to intensify the development of synthetic obsessions. Once the indulgence cycle is under way, we may become aroused and anxious each time the thought intrudes when we are suppressing; but when we let go and think it, the nervousness is overwhelming because we have never allowed ourselves to get used to the idea. The thought that we most want to avoid becomes, in a sense, our greatest fear, and we find ourselves severely agitated in both body and mind whenever it appears.

An Invisible Process.   When we get an obsession it seems to pop into our heads all of a sudden. There is little awareness of any gradual or stepwise pattern of development, and the obsessive thought instead explodes into view. In fact, it is remarkable just how impervious the process is to our scrutiny. If intrusive and troubling unwanted thoughts do become more frequent primarily as a result of the "synthesis" process, it is probably the case that we have experienced several cycles of indulgence of any thought before it breaks into our minds as a truly disturbing vision. We have seen the thought before, in a less disturbing form, and we have suppressed it before as well. Why don't we know that we are doing this to ourselves?

Our lack of awareness may be almost a part of the process. Just as we spend much energy trying to suppress a given thought, we may actively set aside any attempts to come to grips with the mental processes that govern the suppression and the eventual obsession. We ignore these cycles in their early stages because we quickly see that they are linked to the unwanted thought. The schoolgirl with romantic thoughts of her priest thinks only about getting rid of them when she is tempted to reveal her secret, not about how the thoughts have multiplied. Later, she may be surprised at the strength of her single-minded desire. Thus, it may only seem that the obsession enters our minds full-blown. When the obsession was being formed, we were suppressing our attempts to suppress as much as we were suppressing the thought itself.

In essence, we are fooled by our attention to the thought. We believe the *thought* is the problem, we notice when we have the *thought,* and we do our best to get rid of the *thought.* We don't notice, though, that we are in the meantime doing something to the thought. We fail to notice our own attempts to suppress, our own desire to struggle against the thought. So we miss out on at least half of what it means to have an "unwanted thought."

We see the thought, but we are blind to the power of our desire to suppress it. But to miss our own contribution to this is to ignore the only part of the process that we can do something about. We are ignoring the possibility that the suppression is the root of the problem.

Think about it for a minute. In order to have a rebound—a resurgence of an unwanted thought—one must have suppressed the thought first. And in order to synthesize a severe obsession, one must experience a rebound following a thought suppression at least once, and perhaps many times. What this means is that the development of a synthetic obsession is totally dependent on suppression as the first step. We may not understand this as it is happening because we are so busy suppressing. But the thought is not the problem—it is the suppression.

Now, of course there are unwanted thoughts that come *before* suppression. The obsessions we develop from traumas, for instance, are clearly there prior to our desires for avoidance. The ruminations we may have that recall past traumas, then, are often suppressed after they occur. But when no obvious trauma is present, there is the good possibility that the obsession has crept up on us slowly, synthesized over time by a series of our own acts of suppression. The curious fact is that as this process continues, the villain in it all—the desire to suppress—becomes stronger and stronger. Suppression creates the difficulty in the first place, and then continues to grow from it.

Some psychologists have thought that the way to solve all this, to knock out obsessions once and for all, is to help people suppress. They invented a style of therapy known as "thought stopping," in which the therapist calls out "Stop!" whenever the client reports having an unwanted obsessive thought.[170] The client is then encouraged to do the same, at least during the therapy session, and then later to say this silently whenever the obsession returns. Some practitioners have gone so far as to instruct clients to punish themselves for unwanted thoughts, snapping rubber bands on their wrists or pinching themselves.

And as it turns out, this style of "therapy" is a resounding failure.[171] Adding to a person's existing motivation to suppress does not seem to quell unwanted thought.

Freud helped, in his own way, to obscure this fact from psychologists. He was so convinced of the power of repression, the unconscious forgetting of painful thoughts, that he led us to believe that we all get rid of our unwanted thoughts quickly and with little effort. He said we just forget. As it turns out, though, our memories are independent of our wills. It is not so easy to forget. We must constantly concern ourselves with keeping unwanted thoughts out of our minds. Rather than obliterating unwanted thoughts with an all-out attack, we carry out an interminable guerrilla war with these enemies, pushing them back, and back, and back again. Some form of thought suppression is needed all the time to keep the enemy from the gates once we have decided a thought is unwanted.

The price we pay for this mental turmoil is dear. For as it happens, we find that our act of suppressing can make some thoughts into far more daunting enemies than they were when we began. It is as though our suppression feeds them, makes them over into the very problems we were most wanting to avoid. The fact that we often don't notice this until it is too late only attests further to the significant mental efforts we must expend in the pursuit of suppression. We are so busy suppressing, we don't realize that we are often creating our own worst nightmares.

Stop Stopping. The solution at this point should be clear. In many cases of unwanted thought, it may be best to stop suppressing. Admittedly, this is just about the last thing you may want to do, but it may be the best. We have seen that in the case of traumatic obsessions, the major theories suggest that facing up to the trauma may be beneficial. This may not always be the case, and there is certainly a time during and right after the trauma in which one can only wish the thought away. But in general, thinking about it may help. Now, in the case of synthetic obsession, we discover the same rule—and here it is even more evident. Synthetic obsession is *caused* by the suppression, and there is thus no mistaking the proper treatment.

It appears that evidence from a wide array of sources, from many lines of argument, and relevant to a number of specific problems, comes together to suggest that we should think the unthinkable. We should go ahead and think our unwanted thoughts. We should relax our mental control, ironically, because this is the circuitous path we must take to regain it. Even though suppression may seem to be the solution, the only rational response to the thoughts we cry out to avoid, it in fact is the problem, the invisible ogre that can make our own thoughts foreign to us.

The idea that our unwanted thoughts might be good for us is confusing. It is almost as though we were prescribing the disease as a cure for itself, and asking the patient to throw away the medicine. But this approach has a successful history as a therapeutic technique. Victor Frankl was the first to voice the idea clearly in what he called the therapy of "paradoxical intention."[172] He suggested that the way to get rid of unwanted thoughts (or emotions or behaviors), paradoxically, was to invite them in. He reasoned that if people accepted their unacceptable thoughts, they might begin to understand the meaning of these things, and thus relax their overwhelming desire to suppress. This, he felt, would lead to the eventual disappearance of the obsession.

The paradoxical style of therapy appears to be genuinely useful. In one early study, for instance, a number of people who had suffered for years from truly distressing obsessional thoughts were given paradoxical instructions.[173] One patient who had long feared going insane and who thought about this incessantly, for example, was encouraged to drop any attempt to suppress, and instead to elaborate the thought, exaggerate it, and dwell on it deliberately. He was asked to tell himself: "It is true, I am going insane, slowly but surely. I am developing many crazy thoughts and habits. I will be admitted to a mental hospital, put into a straight-jacket and will remain there neglected by everybody until I die. I won't even remember my name. I will forget that I was married and had children, and will become a zombie. I will neglect my appearance and eat like an animal."[174]

The researchers found that "prescribing the disease" actually worked. A substantial number of their clients improved over the course of six weeks of this treatment. Those who did not improve, it turned out, were most often those who found themselves unable to accept the therapeutic suggestion. In other words, some people decided it was just too awful to concentrate attention on their unwanted thought, and so they never went ahead with the advised program of thinking their thought to the hilt. So, in the case of very severe obsessions, it appears that relaxing the suppression can be a useful approach.

This is also true with less severe cases, the "normal obsessions" we all get from time to time. Research on people who report that they worry too much, for instance, has found that a paradoxical approach is successful.[175] These people were asked to arrange for a half-hour worry period at the same time and place every day. Then, whenever they caught themselves worrying outside this time, they were not to suppress the worry, but instead were to make a special point of focusing on it in the worry period. During the worry period, then, they were instructed to do nothing but worry. Over the course of only a four-week treatment program, these people showed a dramatic improvement as compared with another group of worriers who were left untreated. They worried less all day, and they even found they sometimes had nothing to do in the worry period. Although it may not always work, this method is one way to try overcoming worries or other unwanted thoughts.

The reversal of suppression is also a part of the therapy plan that psychologists often use for phobias.[176] Normally, the phobic person scrambles like a cat held against its will whenever the phobic object is near, and this avoidance effectively produces thought suppression as well. But when phobic patients are forced, in small steps, to confront whatever it is they fear, they usually improve dramatically. They may be urged to think about their feared object, or even to encounter it directly. As discussed earlier, this technique has been called "implosive therapy" or "flooding," and it has a particularly good record when it is combined with relaxation suggestions. The relaxation helps the client to go on with the therapy, as it acts to dissipate the anxious symptoms that naturally are aroused. Without being coaxed to approach the feared object, people are motivated by their anxiety to nurse their fears and suppress thoughts about them—and so never can improve.

Why does reversing suppression work? Some theorists say that when we look at our unwanted thoughts closely and turn them all around, we will finally be able to fit their meaning into our lives. This was Frankl's view, and it is shared by many.[177] The idea is that understanding our problems, thinking them through, and finding out how they are linked to all our other thoughts is our common and natural approach to most of life's challenges. The tendency to suppress a thought gets in the way of this, and so blocks us from achieving a meaningful life. There is some part of us that we don't understand, or refuse to understand, and until this is fully resolved, we will not have peace.

Other theories suggest that thinking unwanted thoughts helps us to get rid of them because we are released from emotional or social inhibition. We get better when we confess our problems to others and eliminate the burden of holding back. It may be that we have some emotional reaction to the unwanted thought that in fact might best be expressed; thinking the thought allows the emotion finally to surface. On the other hand, confession may be good for us simply because the very act of inhibiting ourselves from telling others about an unwanted thought has always been the problem. Focusing on the unwanted thought and thinking it may allow us free and easy communication with others about what was formerly a taboo topic.[178]

It may also be the case that confronting an unwanted thought gives us some experience with it, and that this is what makes it less mesmerizing. When we sit and ponder the unwanted thought, we merely get used to it, or as psychologists say, we habituate. We can even become bored with it as we do with most anything that we concentrate on for some time. After all, we can overcome many phobias by allowing ourselves to be exposed to the feared object. We learn that we can "handle it" and the horror disappears. Simple exposure may eliminate our fears by replacing them with the recognition that we are in the presence of normal, usual, and uninteresting things.[179]

Many events that happen once we face an unwanted thought, in short, can be helpful and useful. We may find meaning in our lives, we may be able finally to confess our thoughts to others, we may become habituated to the thought, and we may learn that we are capable of dealing with it. The key to all of these benefits, however, is the basic recognition that the suppression must stop. Once we begin to accept our thoughts, we can gain much more than the obliviousness we seek in suppression. In a way, suppression is required for the existence of obsession. Once we stop suppressing, by definition, we no longer have thoughts we do not want.

This step, of course, is not easy. Deciding to accept and think a thought that we have been running from for days or years is not likely to be an effortless undertaking. But it will probably require no more willpower, no more exertion, than all the work we've put into suppression itself. Turning off the suppression, thinking about the thought, is thus the ultimate act of mental control. In embracing our unwanted thoughts, we escape the tyranny that suppression can hold over us. We no longer must worry about our worries, no longer wish our thoughts away, no longer believe that we are plagued by images that we cannot overcome. When we turn toward these things and look at them closely, they can disappear.

Unwanted thoughts, in many cases, arise from unwanted realities. When we cannot change our realities, we turn to our minds and hope that we can control what goes on there from the inside. But this control process is a swindler, a charlatan that runs off with our minds and gives us nothing in return. The suppression we crave does not save us, and instead can energize the obsessions we wish to avoid. When all around us reality doesn't seem that bad, and yet we live in a world of mental turmoil and despair, the problem may be only that we think we have a problem. If we can bring ourselves to want our unwanted thoughts, we will soon not even notice them.

Ultimately, then, the most important decision we face about mental control is when to use it and when to relax it. There are many thoughts in life that must be suppressed or otherwise sidestepped if we are going to be healthy and moral individuals. We really shouldn't think of hurting others or ourselves, for example, and we shouldn't think of things that will make us forever unhappy. But the impulse to suppress such thoughts is often very natural and easy to accept, a proper plan for what we ought to do. This makes detecting the cases in which suppression is ineffective or harmful doubly difficult. When suppression seems the quick, the easy, the obvious solution to a problem, it may not always be quite so simple. In fact, it may be that our easy solution quickly escalates into an all-out struggle. Thought suppression is a special, potentially dangerous tool in our bag of mental tricks—a tool that must be used, but must be used wisely.

When we try not to think of a white bear, after all, it seems we are just playing a simple game. This thought is surely something we can stop in a moment, we think to ourselves, and so we give it a try. All too soon we find, though, that it won't go away so easily. We try again. And it comes back again. If only we could realize that it will go away only when we welcome it back. It is only then that, like any child with a toy, we will soon tire of dragging it around with us and lose track of it quite naturally.

NOTES

1. Wegner, D. M., Schneider, D. J., Carter, S., III, & White, T. (1987). Paradoxical effects of thought suppression. *Journal of Personality and Social Psychology, 53,* 5–13.

2. *Time,* April 18, 1988, p. 33.

3. Berry, C. S. (1916–1917). Obsessions of normal minds. *Journal of Abnormal Psychology, 11,* 1922.

4. Shackelford, S., & Wegner, D. M. (1985). [Perceived characteristics of unwanted thoughts.] Unpublished research data, Trinity University.

5. Rachman, S., & de Silva, P. (1978). Abnormal and normal obsessions. *Behavioral Research and Therapy, 16,* 233–248.

6. For example, see Freud, S. (1957). Repression. In J. Strachey (Ed.), *The Standard Edition of the Complete Psychological Works of Sigmund Freud* (Vol. 14, pp. 146–158). London: Hogarth. (Original work published 1915.)

7. See Erdelyi, M. H., & Goldberg, B. (1979). Let's not sweep repression under the rug: Toward a cognitive psychology of repression. In J. F. Kihlstrom & F. J. Evans (Eds.), *Functional Disorders of Memory* (pp. 355–402). Hillsdale, NJ: Erlbaum. Also see Holmes, D. S. (1974). Investigation of repression: Differential recall of material experimentally or naturally associated with ego threat. *Psychological Bulletin, 81,* 632–653.

8. Cases of amnesia resemble cases in which people are instructed to forget something during hypnosis, and in both instances real memory loss occurs. See Kihlstrom, J. F. (1983). Instructed forgetting: Hypnotic and nonhypnotic. *Journal of Experimental Psychology: General, 112,* 73–79.

9. Freud, S. (1958). Remembering, repeating, and working through. In J. Strachey (Ed.), *The Standard Edition of the Complete Psychological Works of Sigmund Freud* (Vol. 12, pp. 145–150). London: Hogarth. (Original work published 1914.)

10. Lindemann, E. (1944). Symptomatology and management of acute grief. *American Journal of Psychiatry, 101,* 141–148.

11. Janis, I. L. (1983). Preventing pathogenic denial by means of stress inoculation. In S. Breznitz (Ed.), *The Denial of Stress* (pp. 35–76). New York: International Universities Press.

12. Silver, R. L., Boon, C., & Stones, M. H. (1983). Searching for meaning in misfortune: Making sense of incest. *Journal of Social Issues, 39,* 81–102.

13. Polivy, J., & Herman, C. P. (1985). Dieting and binging: A causal analysis. *American Psychologist, 40,* 193–201.

14. Pennebaker, J. W. (1985). Inhibition and cognition: Toward an understanding of trauma and disease. *Canadian Psychology, 26,* 82–95.

15. James, W. (1890). *Principles of Psychology.* New York: Holt.

16. See Bargh, J. A. (1984). Automatic and conscious processing of social information. In R. S. Wyer, Jr., & T. K. Srull (Eds.), *Handbook of Social Cognition* (Vol. 3, pp. 1–43). Hillsdale, NJ: Erlbaum. Also informative is the basic work of Posner, M. I., & Snyder, C. R. R. (1975). Attention and cognitive control. In R. L. Solso (Ed.), *Information Processing and Cognition: The Loyola Symposium.* Hillsdale, NJ: Erlbaum. There are also a number of useful new perspectives on the automaticity of thought in J. S. Uleman & J. A. Bargh (Eds.) (in press), *Unintended Thought: The Limits of Awareness, Intention, and Control.* New York: Guilford Press.

17. John Dewey (1922). *Human Nature and Conduct* (pp. 28, 29). New York: Holt.

18. Norcross, J. C., Ratzin, A. C., & Payne, D. (in press). Ringing in the New Year: The change processes and reported outcomes of resolutions. *Addictive Behaviors.*

19. See, for instance, the discussion of this by Paul J. Griffiths (1986). *On Being Mindless: Buddhist Meditation and the Mind-Body Problem.* La Salle, IL: Open Court.

20. Rozin, P., Millman, L., & Nemeroff, C. (1986). Operation of the laws of sympathetic magic in disgust and other domains. *Journal of Personality and Social Psychology, 50,* 703–712.

21. This list, translated from Janet, and an interesting discussion of the contents of obsessions are in Reed, G. F. (1985), *Obsessional Experience and Compulsive Behavior.* Orlando, FL: Academic Press.

22. These categories include those from Reed (above), and also ones discussed by Akhtar, S., Wig, N. H., Verma, V. K., Pershod, D., & Verma, S. K. (1975). A phenomenological analysis of symptoms in

obsessive-compulsive neurosis. *British Journal of Psychiatry, 127,* 342–348, and by Rachman, S. J., & Hodgson, R. J. (1980). *Obsessions and Compulsions.* Englewood Cliffs, NJ: Prentice-Hall.

23. Two samples of a total of 128 subjects were studied by Shackelford, S., & Wegner, D. M. (1984). Unwanted thoughts. Unpublished manuscript, Trinity University. The third, which surveyed 75 student subjects, was Frontman, K. (1986). Effects of cognitive strategies in controlling unwanted thoughts. M.A. thesis, Trinity University.

24. Rachman, S., & de Silva, P. (1978). Abnormal and normal obsessions. *Behavior Research and Therapy, 16,* 233–248.

25. A good introduction is given by Freud himself in Freud, S. (1977). *An Outline of Psychoanalysis.* New York: Norton. (Originally published 1917.)

26. A clear and engaging review of current evidence on Freud's ideas is Erdelyi, M. H. (1985). *Psychoanalysis: Freud's Cognitive Psychology.* New York: Freeman.

27. William James's ideas about the kind of trance we get into when we have only one thought are nicely developed in Eugene Taylor's (1983) *William James on Exceptional Mental States.* Amherst: University of Massachusetts Press.

28. James in the Taylor book noted above, p. 8.

29. Minsky, M. (1987). *Society of Mind.* New York: Simon and Schuster.

30. Freud, S. (1960). Jokes and their relation to the unconscious. In J. Strachey (Ed.), *The Standard Edition of the Complete Psychological Works of Sigmund Freud* (Vol. 8). London: Hogarth. (Original work published 1905.)

31. Polivy, J., & Herman, C. P. (1985). Dieting and binging: A causal analysis. *American Psychologist, 40,* 193–201.

32. Keys, A., Brozek, J., Henschel, A., Mickelson, O., & Taylor, H. L. (1950). *The Biology of Human Starvation.* Minneapolis: University of Minnesota Press.

33. Herman, C. P., & Mack, D. (1975). Restrained and unrestrained eating. *Journal of Personality, 43,* 647–660. Much of the work in this area is put into practical suggestions by Polivy, J., & Herman, C. P. (1983). *Breaking the Diet Habit.* New York: Basic Books.

34. Jordan, A., & Wegner, D. M. (1987). Obsessive thinking about smoking after impromptu self-control. Paper presented at the meeting of the Midwestern Psychological Association, Chicago.

35. Marlatt, G. P., & Parks, G. A. (1982). Self-management of

addictive behaviors. In P. Karoly & F. H. Kanfer (Eds.), *Self-Management and Behavior Change* (pp. 443–488). New York: Pergamon Press.

36. John Dewey (1922). *Human Nature and Conduct* (pp. 34–35). New York: Holt.

37. An absorbing discussion of lies and their detection is in Ekman, P. (1985). *Telling Lies.* New York: Norton.

38. The problem of social stigmatization is treated in depth by Jones, E. E., Farina, A., Hastorf, A. H., Markus, H., Miller, D. T., & Scott, R. A. (1984). *Social Stigma: The Psychology of Marked Relationships.* New York: Freeman.

39. Pennebaker, J. W. (1985). Inhibition and cognition: Toward an understanding of trauma and disease. *Canadian Psychology, 26,* 82–95. Also, see Pennebaker, J. W. (in press). Confession and health. In S. Fisher & J. Reason (Eds.), *Handbook of Life Stress, Cognition, and Health.* Chichester, Eng.: Wiley.

40. Rachman, S. (1980). Emotional processing. *Behaviour Research and Therapy, 18,* 51–60.

41. Two particularly fine examples of this are Braitenberg, N. (1984). *Vehicles.* Cambridge, MA: MIT Press, and Minsky, M. (1987). *Society of Mind.* Cambridge, MA: MIT Press.

42. Jack Nicholson's character in *The Shining* did something like this. His wife thought he was working on a novel, and instead he was typing, over and over, "All work and no play makes Jack a dull boy." Her discovery of the manuscript, hundreds of pages of it, was one of the most striking revelations of madness ever in film.

43. Douglas Hofstadter has written broadly and elegantly on the problem of self-reference, both mental and in symbol systems generally. The entire text of his 1979 book, *Gödel, Escher, Bach: The Eternal Golden Braid* (New York: Basic Books), is relevant to this, but his essay on self-referent sentences is particularly telling: Chapter 1 in Hofstadter, D. (1985). *Metamagical Themas.* New York: Basic Books.

44. This bit of history is from an interesting collection of paradox lore: Quine, W. V. (April 1962). Paradox. *Scientific American, 206,* 84–96.

45. Russell, B. *Introduction to Mathematical Philosophy* (p. 135). New York: Simon and Schuster.

46. You can prove this by repeating Russell's class/member logic with thoughts about thoughts. Just use the same trick he did, but instead of envisioning a class that is not a member of itself, imagine a thought that is not about itself. If one then thinks about this thought

that is not about itself, one can ask if *this* thought is about itself. If it is, then it is about a thought that is not about itself, so it is not. If it is not, then it is about a thought that is about itself, so it is.

47. Tarski, A. (June 1969). Truth and proof. *Scientific American,* *220,* 63–77.

48. Miller, G. A. (1956). The magical number seven, plus or minus two: Some limits on our capacity for processing information. *Psychological Review, 63,* 81–97.

49. For example, Anderson, J. R., & Bower, G. H. (1973). *Human Associative Memory.* Washington, D. C.: V. H. Winston.

50. Much interesting research has been directed to the problem of how much we know about our own mental processes as they occur. It turns out we don't know all that much sometimes. The best example of this is when we have a "creative insight" and it feels as though it just drops from the sky into our heads. Some fine leads on this topic are in Nisbett, R. E., & Wilson, T. D. (1977). Telling more than we can know: Verbal reports on mental processes. *Psychological Review, 84,* 231–259. Also, see Klatzky, R. L. (1984). *Memory and Awareness.* New York: Freeman.

51. Shallice, T. (1978). The dominant action system. In K. S. Pope & J. L. Singer (Eds.), *The Stream of Consciousness* (pp. 115–157). New York: Plenum.

52. Evidence for these kinds of automatic thought processes is given by Nisbett and Wilson and by Klatzky (noted above), and also in a wide variety of the writings of cognitive psychologists. Good examples are in Dixon, N. (1981). *Preconscious Processing.* New York: Wiley. Also, see Bowers, K. S., & Meichenbaum, D. (1985) (Eds.). *The Unconscious Reconsidered.* New York: Wiley.

53. Hasher, L., & Zacks, R. T. (1979). Automatic and effortful processes in memory. *Journal of Experimental Psychology: General, 108,* 356–388.

54. One theory of action holds that whenever people finish doing something successfully, they immediately turn to thinking of why or with what consequence they did it—see Vallacher, R. R., & Wegner, D. M. (1985). *A Theory of Action Identification.* Hillsdale, NJ: Erlbaum. If this is true, then whenever one thinks successfully of Y, there will be a natural tendency to move back to the intended consequence of this (avoiding X), and so to remind oneself again of X. I thank Daniel Gilbert for pointing out this connection to me.

55. Rachman, S., & de Silva, P. (1978). Normal and abnormal obsessions. *Behavior Research and Therapy, 16,* 233–248. Also relevant is the finding that most people prefer distraction to any other

mental strategy for coping with pain; see McCaul, K. D., & Haugvedt, C. (1982). Attention, distraction, and cold pressor pain. *Journal of Personality and Social Psychology, 43,* 154–162.

56. Borkovec, T. D., Robinson, E., Pruzinsky, T., & DePree, J. A. (1983). Preliminary exploration of worry: Some characteristics and processes. *Behavioral Research and Therapy, 21,* 9–16.

57. McCaul, K. D., & Malott, J. M. (1984). Distraction and coping with pain. *Psychological Bulletin, 95,* 516–533.

58. Corah, N. L., Gale, E. N., & Illig, S. J. (1979). The use of relaxation and distraction to reduce psychological stress during dental procedures. *Journal of Dental Research, 58,* 1347–1351. Corah, N. L., Gale, E. N., Pace, L. F., & Seyrek, S. K. (1981). Relaxation and musical programming as means of reducing psychological stress during dental procedures. *Journal of the American Dental Association, 103,* 232–234.

59. Westcott, T. B., & Horan, J. J. (1977). The effects of anger and relaxation forms of in vivo emotive imagery on pain tolerance. *Canadian Journal of Behavioral Science, 9,* 216–223.

60. Margaret Atwood (1985). *The Handmaid's Tale* (p. 251). New York: Ballantine.

61. Brucato, D. B. (1978). The psychological control of pain. Unpublished doctoral dissertation, Kent State University. Cited in McCaul & Malott (1984), noted above.

62. Leventhal, H., Shacham, S., Boothe, L. S., & Leventhal, E. (1981). The role of attention in distress and control during childbirth. Unpublished manuscript, University of Wisconsin, Madison. See also Leventhal, H., Brown, D., Shacham, S., & Engquist, G. (1979). The effects of preparatory information about sensations, threat of pain, and attention on cold pressor distress. *Journal of Personality and Social Psychology, 37,* 688–714.

63. McCaul & Malott (1984), noted above.

64. Wegner, D. M., Schneider, D. J., Carter, S. R., III, & White, T. L. (1987). Paradoxical effects of thought suppression. *Journal of Personality and Social Psychology, 53,* 5–13. (Experiment 2)

65. The flow theory is by Csikszentmihalyi, M. (1975). *Beyond Boredom and Anxiety.* San Francisco: Jossey-Bass.

66. There is a detailed discussion of this in Vallacher, R. R., & Wegner, D. M. (1985). *A Theory of Action Identification.* Hillsdale, NJ: Erlbaum.

67. This was a study conducted by Duval, Wicklund, and Fine cited in Duval, S., & Wicklund, R. A. (1972). *A Theory of Objective Self Awareness.* New York: Academic Press.

68. Gibbons, F. X., & Wicklund, R. A. (1976). Selective exposure to self. *Journal of Research in Personality, 10,* 98–106.

69. Wegner, D. M., & Schaefer, D. (1978). The concentration of responsibility: An objective self awareness analysis of group size effects in helping situations. *Journal of Personality and Social Psychology, 36,* 147–155.

70. Roy Baumeister has argued, for example, that sexual masochism is often caused by a motive to avoid thinking about oneself, one's identity, and one's characteristics. This doesn't mean that self-distraction always yields masochism, only that strange and potentially harmful activities can follow when, rather than pursuing our interests, we are escaping our disinterests. See Baumeister, R. F. (1988). Masochism as escape from self. *Journal of Sex Research, 25,* 28–59.

71. Arendt, H. (1963). *Eichmann in Jerusalem: A Report on the Banality of Evil.* New York: Viking.

72. In Arendt, noted above, p. 46.

73. Mullen, B., & Suls, J. (1982). The effectiveness of attention and rejection as coping styles: A meta-analysis of temporal differences. *Journal of Psychosomatic Research, 26,* 43–49. Also, see Suls, J., & Fletcher, B. (1985). The relative efficacy of avoidant and nonavoidant coping strategies: A meta-analysis. *Health Psychology, 4,* 249–288.

74. My friend Chris Gilbert once wrote an enchanting science fiction story about a boy who dabbled in his father's biofeedback lab and began to learn how to control his various bodily functions—his heart rate, blood pressure, and so on. The twist in the story was that the boy eventually had to maintain conscious control over these things to keep them going. The stress due to having to remember each heartbeat, not to mention the operation of every other organ, became too much to bear and he thought he would lose his life. Finally, and fortunately, he lost consciousness—and all the automatic processes could thus take over once again to save him. See Gilbert, C. (May 1984). Veils of the body. *Amazing,* pp. 58–70.

75. DePaulo, B. M., Lanier, K., & Davis, T. (1983). Detecting the deceit of the motivated liar. *Journal of Personality and Social Psychology, 45,* 1096–1103.

76. Tesser, A., & Moore, J. (1986). On the convergence of public and private aspects of self. In R. Baumeister (Ed.), *Public Self and Private Self* (pp. 99–116). New York: Springer-Verlag.

77. Gilbert, D. T., Krull, D. S., & Pelham, B. W. (1987). Of thoughts unspoken: Behavioral inhibition and social inference. *Journal of Personality and Social Psychology, 55,* 685–694. A series of studies on this topic is presented in Gilbert, D. T. (in press). Thinking lightly

about others: Automatic components of the social inference process. In J. S. Uleman & J. A. Bargh (Eds.), *Unintended Thought: The Limits of Awareness, Intention, and Control.* New York: Guilford Press.

78. Behavior therapists refer to this as a "stimulus control" strategy for the self-control of behavior. They note that animals of all kinds will often do something only with the right stimulus—say, a dog will roll over only when you say "roll over." That stimulus, then, has control over the behavior. See, e.g., Kanfer, F. H. (1980). Self-management methods. In F. H. Kanfer & A. P. Goldstein (Eds.), *Helping People Change: A Textbook of Methods* (pp. 334–389). New York: Pergamon Press.

79. Albert, S. (1977). Temporal comparison theory. *Psychological Review, 84,* 485–503.

80. It is worth noting that the absence of a close partner can reduce our abilities to remember many things. Just as circumstances can cue memories of the partner, the partner can be a cue to lots of thoughts. When the partner is gone these thoughts may become inaccessible. See the comments on this in Wegner, D. M., Giuliano, T., & Hertel, P. T. (1985). Cognitive interdependence in close relationships. In W. Ickes (Ed.), *Compatible and Incompatible Relationships* (pp. 253–276). New York: Springer-Verlag.

81. Hertel, P. T. (1987). Monitoring external memory. Paper presented at the Conference on Practical Aspects of Memory, Swansea, Wales.

82. Anderson, J. R., & Reder, L. (1979). Elaborative processing explanation of depth of processing. In L. S. Cermak & F. I. M. Craik (Eds.), *Levels of Processing in Human Memory.* Hillsdale, NJ: Erlbaum.

83. McCall, G. J., & Simmons, J. T. (1978). *Identities and Interaction* (rev. ed.). New York: Free Press. A similar idea, the "plausibility structure," was introduced by Berger, P. L., & Luckmann, T. (1967). *The Social Construction of Reality.* Garden City, NY: Doubleday-Anchor.

84. An engaging explication of this idea is in Swann, W. B., Jr. (1983). Self-verification: Bringing social reality into harmony with the self. In J. Suls & A. G. Greenwald (Eds.), *Psychological Perspectives on the Self* (Vol. 2, pp. 33–66). Hillsdale, NJ: Erlbaum.

85. Wenzlaff, R. M., & Prohaska, M. L. (1987). Depression and the desire to meet others: When misery prefers company. Unpublished manuscript, University of Texas at San Antonio.

86. Wachtel, P. L. (1973). Psychodynamics, behavior therapy, and the implacable experimenter: An inquiry into the consistency of per-

sonality. *Journal of Abnormal Psychology, 82,* 324–334. See also Snyder, M., & Ickes, W. (1985). Personality and social behavior. In G. Lindzey & E. Aronson (Eds.), *Handbook of Social Psychology* (3rd ed., Vol. 2, pp. 883–947). New York: Random House.

87. The idea that we are continually extending ourselves from past to future by creating ecological niches in which our past selves can survive is nicely developed by Hormuth, S. E. (in press). *The Self-Concept and Change: An Ecological Approach.* Cambridge: Cambridge University Press.

88. A clear theoretical account of the scientific literature on this phenomenon is given by Snow, D. A., & Machalek, R. (1983). The convert as a social type. In R. Collins (Ed.), *Sociological Theory* (pp. 259–289). New York: Jossey-Bass.

89. Koestler, A. (1952). *The God that Failed* (p. 19). New York: Crossman.

90. The chapter by Swann noted above contends that resolutions to change are common responses to life crises, circumstances in which one's prior views of self and world seem not to be working. Such crises do not, however, always yield lasting change.

91. More complete details of this are available in Snow and Machalek's chapter noted above.

92. Doughty, W. L. (1955). *John Wesley: Preacher* (p. 57). London: Epworth.

93. Swann, W. B., Jr., & Predmore, S. C. (1985). Intimates as agents of social support: Sources of consolation or despair? *Journal of Personality and Social Psychology, 49,* 1609–1617.

94. They do not appreciate the fact, for example, that they are more inclined to recall something in the same place that they learned it. See Hertel, P. T., Anooshian, L. J., & Ashbrook, P. (1986). The accuracy of beliefs about retrieval cues. *Memory and Cognition, 14,* 265–269.

95. Wegner, D. M., Schneider, D. J., McMahon, S., & Knutson, B. M. (1989). Taking worry out of context: The enhancement of thought suppression effectiveness in new surroundings. Unpublished manuscript, Trinity University.

96. James, W. (1979). *The Will to Believe.* Cambridge, MA: Harvard University Press. (Original work published 1897.)

97. See, for example, the attitude and belief research reviewed by Abelson, R., Aronson, E., McGuire, W. J., Newcomb, T. M., Rosenberg, M. J., & Tannenbaum, P. H. (Eds.) (1968). *Theories of Cognitive Consistency: A Sourcebook.* Chicago: Rand McNally.

98. Wegner, D. M., Wenzlaff, R., Kerker, R. M., & Beattie, A. E.

(1981). Incrimination through innuendo: Can media questions become public answers? *Journal of Personality and Social Psychology, 40,* 822–832.

99. Even Jesus Christ appears to have done this at times. Jay Haley (1986) has made a fascinating account of how Christ used double messages to get his work done in *The Power Tactics of Jesus Christ and Other Essays,* 2nd ed. Rockville, MD: Triangle Press.

100. Bramel, D. A. (1962). A dissonance theory approach to defensive projection. *Journal of Abnormal and Social Psychology, 69,* 121–129.

101. Walster, E., Berscheid, E., Abrahams, D., & Aronson, V. (1967). Effectiveness of debriefing following deception experiments. *Journal of Personality and Social Psychology, 6,* 371–380.

102. Ross, L., Lepper, M. R., & Hubbard, M. (1975). Perseverance in self-perception and social perception: Biased attributional processes in the debriefing paradigm. *Journal of Personality and Social Psychology, 32,* 880–892.

103. Wegner, D. M., Coulton, G., & Wenzlaff, R. (1985). The transparency of denial: Briefing in the debriefing paradigm. *Journal of Personality and Social Psychology, 49,* 338–346.

104. Hirt, E. R., & Sherman, S. J. (1985). The role of prior knowledge in explaining hypothetical events. *Journal of Experimental Social Psychology, 21,* 519–543.

105. Although this was not tested in the Hirt/Sherman experiment noted above, we would also predict that the novice would be highly susceptible to innuendo about a team. So, for instance, if we said "MSU can't possibly win *again,*" the novice would have nothing to think but that Michigan State wins a lot—and so would be swayed by a denial to believe the underlying information, and not the intended falsification.

106. See Snyder, M., & Swann, W. B., Jr. (1978). Hypothesis testing in social interaction. *Journal of Personality and Social Psychology, 36,* 1202–1212. The "not an introvert" experiment was by Snyder, M., & White, P. (1981). Testing hypotheses about other people: Strategies of verification and falsification. *Personality and Social Psychology Bulletin, 7,* 39–43.

107. Another way of talking about this is to say that whatever thought we begin with serves as an "anchor" we will return to. Added thoughts in that area, including denials or attempts at disregarding or ignoring, will then be held in place by that anchor. They thus cannot get very far from it. This notion has a long history in sensory psychology, and has been developed in the area of decision making by

Kahneman, D., & Tversky, A. (1973). On the psychology of prediction. *Psychological Review, 80,* 237–251.

108. Wason, P. C., & Johnson-Laird, P. N. (1972). *Psychology of Reasoning.* Cambridge, MA: Harvard University Press.

109. Gilbert, D. (1989). How mental systems believe. Unpublished manuscript, University of Texas at Austin.

110. In his classic study of the psychology of prejudice, Allport suggests that the first reaction to perceiving the "conflict" of prejudice is to deny it. See Allport, G. W. (1954). *The Nature of Prejudice.* Reading, MA: Addison-Wesley.

111. Fiske, S. T. (in press). Examining the role of intent, toward understanding its role in stereotyping and prejudice. In J. Uleman & J. Bargh (Eds.), *Unintended Thought: The Limits of Awareness, Intention, and Control.* New York: Guilford Press. See also Neuberg, S. L., & Fiske, S. T. (1987). Motivational influences on impression formation: Outcome dependency, accuracy-driven attention, and individuating processes. *Journal of Personality and Social Psychology, 53,* 431–444.

112. Simon, H. A. (1967). Motivational and emotional controls of cognition. *Psychological Review, 74,* 29–39.

113. Spock, the pointy-eared character on "Star Trek," was renowned for having no emotion. This quirk provided a centerpiece for several episodes. What Spock seemed to be missing, however, was not emotion in the sense that Simon describes it. Spock was certainly able to interrupt his ongoing activities and respond to those pesky Klingons. What he lacked was merely emotional expression—the bodily, facial, and experiential components of emotion that allow us and others to know that we are feeling something.

114. Plutchik, R. (1980). *Emotion: A Psychoevolutionary Synthesis.* New York: Harper & Row.

115. Such models have been proposed by Bower, G. H. (1981). Mood and memory. *American Psychologist, 36,* 129–148; and also by Isen, A. M. (1984). Toward understanding the role of affect in cognition. In R. S. Wyer, Jr., & T. K. Srull (Eds.), *Handbook of Social Cognition* (Vol. 3, pp. 179–236). Hillsdale, NJ: Erlbaum.

116. See the Bower paper noted above for several studies of this kind. Even more are reviewed in Blaney, P. H. (1986). Affect and memory: A review. *Psychological Bulletin, 99,* 229–246.

117. Beck, A. T. (1976). *Cognitive Therapy and the Emotional Disorders.* New York: International Universities Press.

118. Dostoevsky, F. (1972). *Notes from Underground* (p. 19). Trans. J. Coulson. New York: Penguin Books. (Original publication, 1864.)

119. Severe depression, on average, tends to lift over the course of about six months. Goodwin, F. K. (1977). Diagnosis of affective disorders. In M. E. Jarvik (Ed.), *Psychopharmacology in the Practice of Medicine* (pp. 219–228). New York: Appleton-Century-Crofts.

120. Some of the central ideas in this form of therapy are described in Kendall, P. C., & Hollon, S. D. (1979). *Cognitive-Behavioral Interventions.* New York: Academic Press. Applying these ideas to yourself is possible as well. Some good suggestions are given by Burns, D. D. (1980). *Feeling Good: The New Mood Therapy.* New York: Morrow; and by Lewinsohn, P. M., Muñoz, R. F., Youngren, M. A., & Zeiss, A. M. (1986). *Control Your Depression.* New York: Prentice-Hall.

121. These are the two most general methods of cognitive therapy; see Goldfried, M. R., & Goldfried, A. P. (1980). Cognitive change methods. In F. H. Kanfer & A. P. Goldstein (Eds.), *Helping People Change: A Textbook of Methods* (pp. 97–130). New York: Pergamon Press.

122. See, for example, Koriat, A., Melkman, R., Averill, J. R., & Lazarus, R. (1972). The self-control of reactions to a stressful film. *Journal of Personality, 40,* 601–619; a more theoretical treatment of this idea is given by Clark, M. S., & Isen, A. M. (1982). Toward understanding the relationship between feeling states and social behavior. In A. H. Hastorf & A. M. Isen (Eds.), *Cognitive Social Psychology* (pp. 73–108). New York: Elsevier/North-Holland; also, see Klinger, E. (1982). On the self-management of mood, affect, and attention. In P. Karoly & F. H. Kanfer (Eds.), *Self-Management and Behavior Change* (pp. 129–164). New York: Pergamon Press.

123. Stanislavski, C. (1965). *An Actor Prepares.* Trans. E. R. Hapgood. New York: Theatre Arts Books. (Originally published 1948.)

124. Turner, S. M., Beidel, D. C., & Nathan, R. S. (1985). Biological factors in obsessive-compulsive disorders. *Psychological Bulletin, 97,* 430–450.

125. Wenzlaff, R. M., Wegner, D. M., & Roper, D. (1988). Depression and mental control: The resurgence of unwanted negative thoughts. *Journal of Personality and Social Psychology 55,* 882–892.

126. Beck, A. T., & Beamesderfer, A. (1974). Assessment of depression: The depression inventory. In P. Pichot (Ed.), *Psychological Measurements in Psychopharmacology. Modern Problems in Pharmacopsychiatry* (Vol. 7). Basel, Switzerland: Darger.

127. All the participants in the research eventually saw both a sad and a happy story, so their emotional experience was balanced somewhat by the time their participation was complete. I've not reprinted

a happy story for you here, so I might mention that the mother in the sad story was actually mistaken. Her baby soon regained consciousness, and later that day everyone went to McDonald's for chocolate shakes.

128. The participants in the study were also asked to make a mark in the margin if they thought of the story. An analysis of the frequency of these marks revealed the same pattern of findings.

129. Meichenbaum, D. (1977). *Cognitive Behavior Modification: An Integrative Approach.* New York: Plenum.

130. Isen, A. M., Shalker, T., Clark, M., & Karp, L. (1978). Affect, accessibility of material in memory and behavior: A cognitive loop? *Journal of Personality and Social Psychology, 36,* 1–12.

131. Bradley, G. W. (1978). Self-serving biases in the attribution process: A reexamination of the fact or fiction question. *Journal of Personality and Social Psychology, 36,* 56–71.

132. Taylor, S. E., & Brown, J. D. (1988). Illusion and well-being: A social psychological perspective on mental health. *Psychological Bulletin, 103,* 193–210.

133. Alloy, L. B., & Abramson, L. Y. (1979). Judgment of contingency in depressed and nondepressed students: Sadder but wiser? *Journal of Experimental Psychology: General, 108,* 441–485.

134. Have you ever noticed that people almost always underestimate how long it will take them to do something? For every appliance I've gotten back from the repair shop early, I've gotten 9 to 12 million late. I'm guilty of this, too, of telling people I'll be there before I can be, or of promising that I'll have a project done before I really can. You would think that just by chance, people would get things done early half the time and late half the time—but we're far more often later than we expected. The belief we will do things quickly may be part of our automatic mood shield. Perhaps if everyone were a bit more depressed, we'd get rid of this epidemic error of judgment.

135. This notion of "dissociation" has a long history in clinical psychology and psychiatry, beginning with the theories of Pierre Janet, and is one of the few reasonable explanations we have for the phenomena of hypnosis and other states in which a person seems unaware consciously of thoughts and behaviors that are evident to others. See Janet, P. (1907). *The Major Symptoms of Hysteria.* New York: Macmillan. More contemporary work along this line is discussed by Kihlstrom, J. (1985). Posthypnotic amnesia and the dissociation of memory. In G. H. Bower (Ed.), *The Psychology of Learning and Motivation* (Vol. 19, pp. 131–178). New York: Academic Press.

136. Reason, J., & Lucas, D. (1984). Using cognitive diaries to in-

vestigate naturally occurring memory blocks. In J. E. Harris & P. E. Morris (Eds.), *Everyday Memory, Actions, and Absentmindedness* (pp. 53–70). London: Academic Press.

137. Fear is usually said to occur in the presence of a realistic danger, whereas anxiety occurs without it. Phobia, in turn, is exaggerated fear. These distinctions and others are developed clearly by Marks, I. M. (1987). *Fears, Phobias, and Rituals: Panic, Anxiety, and their Disorders.* New York: Oxford University Press.

138. Freud, S. (1936). *The Problem of Anxiety.* New York: Norton. (Original work published 1923.)

139. Tests of anxiety typically take the form of symptom checklists or simple reports that one is nervous; see, for example, Taylor, J. A. (1953). A personality scale of manifest anxiety. *Journal of Abnormal and Social Psychology, 48,* 285–290. Tests of neurotic tendencies share this symptom focus as well; see, for example, Eysenck, H. J. (1959). *The Maudsley Personality Inventory.* London: University of London Press. People who report having many physical symptoms also generally report being anxious and nervous; see Pennebaker, J. W. (1982). *The Psychology of Physical Symptoms.* New York: Springer-Verlag.

140. More detail on what these terms mean, and on the nature of bodily responses to psychological events in general, is available in Sternbach, R. A. (1966). *Principles of Psychophysiology.* New York: Academic Press.

141. Although the body can sometimes become upset in this way without the mind's being particularly aware of it, and the mind can occasionally think the body is upset when it really is not, as a rule the self-perception of nervousness corresponds at least roughly to measurable changes in bodily processes. See Pennebaker, noted above, for a more complete discussion of this.

142. Grings, W. W., & Dawson, M. E. (1978). *Emotions and Bodily Responses: A Psychophysiological Approach.* New York: Academic Press.

143. Schachter, S., & Singer, J. (1962). Cognitive, social, and physiological determinants of emotional state. *Psychological Review, 69,* 379–399.

144. You may balk at this theory and insist that emotions are really deeper than this. And in doing this, you are following the reasoning of several researchers who have argued on the basis of different kinds of evidence that emotions are more "wired in" than this labeling perspective would suggest. One argument is that people can have good or bad emotional reactions to things without even being able to recognize consciously what those things are (Zajonc, R. B. [1980]. Feeling

and thinking: Preferences need no inferences. *American Psychologist, 35,* 151–175). Another is that people's self-reports of their feelings can diverge dramatically from their feeling-relevant behaviors such as approach or avoidance (Wilson, T. D. [1985]. Strangers to ourselves: The origins and accuracy of beliefs about one's own mental states. In J. H. Harvey & G. Weary (Eds.), *Attributions in Contemporary Psychology* [pp. 9–36]. New York: Academic Press). A third argument is that the body's arousal is emotion-specific, and that measurably different physiological states accompanying each emotion serve as anchors that determine what each emotion is, despite any changes that come from later relabeling (e.g., Schwartz, G. E., Weinberger, D. A., & Singer, J. A. [1981]. Cardiovascular differentiation of happiness, sadness, anger and fear following imagery and exercise. *Psychosomatic Medicine, 43,* 343–364). These points of view suggest that there are multiple sources of mental and physical information about what emotion we are feeling at any one time, some of which may be activated prior to others. Overall, they suggest it may be worthwhile to pursue arguments on whether one emotion may be more "true" than another.

145. Maslach, C. (1979). Negative emotional biasing of unexplained arousal. *Journal of Personality and Social Psychology, 37,* 953–969.

146. Wegner, D. M., & Giuliano, T. (1980). Arousal-induced attention to self. *Journal of Personality and Social Psychology, 38,* 719–726.

147. Koriat, A., Melkman, R., Averill, J. A., & Lazarus, R. S. (1972). The self-control of emotional reactions to a stressful film. *Journal of Personality, 40,* 601–619.

148. Martin, B. (1964). Expression and inhibition of sex motive arousal in college males. *Journal of Abnormal and Social Psychology, 68,* 307–312.

149. Wegner, D. M., Blake, A., Wu, J., & Page, M. (1989). The suppression of exciting thoughts. Unpublished manuscript, Trinity University.

150. This study established one other key finding: Some subjects in the study were not tape recorded, and they were assured that there was no way in which anyone could hear the exact words they were saying as they verbalized their thoughts. This special group of participants was included to determine whether people were merely nervous during the suppression of sex thoughts because they were embarrassed in anticipation that someone listening to the tape would think they were obsessed with sex when they couldn't stop the thought. As it turned out, even these individuals who were able to speak secretly showed the unusual excitement during the suppression of sex thoughts.

151. There is some evidence that skin conductance levels are heightened by inhibition or suppression alone (Pennebaker, J. W., & Chew, C. H. [1985]. Behavioral inhibition and electrodermal activity during deception. *Journal of Personality and Social Psychology, 49,* 1427–1433), but this was not observed in our studies.

152. Borkovec, T. D. (1974). Heart-rate process during systematic desensitization and implosive therapy for analog anxiety. *Behavior Therapy, 5,* 636–641.

153. Safer, M. A., Tharps, Q. J., Jackson, T. C., & Leventhal, H. (1979). Determinants of three stages of delay in seeking care at a medical clinic. *Medical Care, 17,* 11–29. This study also showed, by the way, that looking up symptoms in a medical book can contribute to delay in deciding that one is ill.

154. Jacobson, E. (1938). *Progressive Relaxation,* 2nd ed. Chicago: University of Chicago Press.

155. Jacobson, as noted above, p. 53.

156. It seems that exercise may serve to protect people against the ill effects that stress can have on their health. An eight-month study of 200 high school girls indicated that those who exercised regularly were less likely to report illness following stresses such as moving or a romantic breakup. Brown, J. D., & Siegel, J. M. (in press). Exercise as a buffer of life stress: A prospective study. *Health Psychology.*

157. Freud, S. (1955). Beyond the pleasure principle. In J. Strachey (Ed.), *The Standard Edition of the Complete Psychological Works of Sigmund Freud* (Vol. 18). London: Hogarth. (Original work published 1920.)

158. See, e.g., Ellis, E. M. (1983). A review of empirical rape research: Victim reactions and response to treatment. *Clinical Psychology Review, 3,* 473–490.

159. Silver, R. L., Boon, C., & Stones, M. H. (1983). Searching for meaning in misfortune: Making sense of incest. *Journal of Social Issues, 39,* 81–102.

160. Lehman, D. R., Wortman, C. B., & Williams, A. F. (1987). Long-term effects of losing a spouse or child in a motor vehicle crash. *Journal of Personality and Social Psychology, 52,* 218–231.

161. Ayalon, O. (1983). Coping with terrorism: The Israeli case. In D. J. Meichenbaum & M. E. Jaremko (Eds.), *Stress Reduction and Prevention,* (pp. 293–339). New York: Plenum.

162. See, e.g., DeFazio, V. J., Rustin, S., & Diamond, A. (1975). Symptom development in Vietnam era veterans. *Journal of Contemporary Psychotherapy, 7,* 9–15.

163. This is consistent with the notion that emotional ideas in mem-

ory may be more general or basic than cognitive ones. It is supported by the finding, for instance, that we remember better those neutral things we have been called on to evaluate or show emotion toward than the ones we have viewed only with detachment. See Hyde, T. W., & Jenkins, J. J. (1969). The differential effects of incidental tasks on the organization of recall of a list of highly associated words. *Journal of Experimental Psychology, 82,* 472–481. This argument is developed more fully by Zajonc, R. B. (1980). Feeling and thinking: Preferences need no inferences. *American Psychologist, 35,* 151–175.

164. Breuer, J., & Freud, S. (1955). *Studies on Hysteria.* In J. Strachey (Ed.), *The Standard Edition of the Complete Psychological Works of Sigmund Freud,* Vol. 2. London: Hogarth. (Original work published 1895.) The more modern works reflecting this idea include Rachman, S. (1980). Emotional processing. *Behaviour Research and Therapy, 18,* 51–60; Foa, E. B., & Kozak, M. J. (1986). Emotional processing of fear: Exposure to corrective information. *Psychological Bulletin, 99,* 20–35.

165. This argument is put forward most clearly by Epstein, S. (1983). Natural healing processes of the mind: Graded stress inoculation as an inherent coping mechanism. In D. Meichenbaum & M. E. Jaremko (Eds.), *Stress Reduction and Prevention* (pp. 39–66). New York: Plenum. However, the idea that obsession is part of a coping process is also suggested by the observation that victims may be thinking repeatedly of the events in trying to find meaning or goal satisfaction in their traumas. The self-healing process is thus part of the theories suggested by Silver, Boon, & Stones, noted earlier, and by Martin, L., & Tesser, A. (in press). Toward a general model of ruminative thought. In J. S. Uleman & J. A. Bargh (Eds.), *Unintended Thought: The Limits of Awareness, Intention, and Control.* New York: Guilford Press.

166. Horowitz, M. (1975). Intrusive and repetitive thoughts after experimental stress. *Archives of General Psychiatry, 32,* 1457–1463.

167. Wetzler, S. E., & Sweeney, J. A. (1986). Childhood amnesia: An empirical demonstration. In D. C. Rubin (Ed.), *Autobiographical Memory* (pp. 191–201). Cambridge: Cambridge University Press.

168. A particularly elegant version of this theory is suggested by Jacobs, W. J., & Nadel, L. (1985). Stress-induced recovery of fears and phobias. *Psychological Review, 92,* 512–531.

169. The nature of feedback processes in systems of all kinds is developed by Bertalanffy, L. von (1968). *General System Theory.* New York: Braziller. Clear descriptions of how they work in human behavior are found in Powers, W. T. (1973). *Behavior: The Control of Perception.* Chicago: Aldine, and in Carver, C. S., & Scheier, M. F.

(1981). *Attention and Self-Regulation: A Control-Theory Approach to Human Behavior*. New York: Springer-Verlag.

170. Wolpe, J., & Lazarus, A. A. (1966). *Behavior Therapy Techniques*. New York: Pergamon Press.

171. One summary of the studies of thought stopping indicates that it appears no better than doing nothing at all (Reed, G. F. [1985]. *Obsessional Experience and Compulsive Behavior*. Orlando, FL: Academic Press).

172. Frankl, V. (1960). Paradoxical intention: A logotherapeutic technique. *American Journal of Psychotherapy, 14,* 520–525.

173. Solyom, L., Garza-Perez, J., Ledwidge, B. L., & Solyom, C. (1972). Paradoxical intention in the treatment of obsessive thoughts: A pilot study. *Comprehensive Psychiatry, 13,* 291–297.

174. From Solyom and colleagues noted above, p. 293.

175. Borkovec, T. D., Wilkinson, L., Folensbee, R., & Lerman, C. (1983). Stimulus control applications to the treatment of worry. *Behaviour Research and Therapy, 21,* 247–251.

176. See, for example, Morris, R. J. (1980). Fear reduction methods. In F. H. Kanfer & A. P. Goldstein (Eds.), *Helping People Change* (pp. 248–293). New York: Pergamon Press.

177. Most notably, the recent work of Roxane Silver exemplifies this approach. Her paper with Boon and Stones is a classic in this area. It is noted above.

178. James Pennebaker's work is most central to this idea. His studies show that confessing our problems and traumas to others will release the burden of inhibition, and so render us less likely to obsess. See Pennebaker, J. W. (1985). Inhibition and cognition: Toward an understanding of trauma and disease. *Canadian Psychology, 26,* 82–95.

179. Foa, E. B., & Kozak, M. J. (1986). Emotional processing of fear: Exposure to corrective information. *Psychological Bulletin, 99,* 20–35.

INDEX

Miller, George A., 50, 56, 185
Millman, L., 182
Minsky, Marvin, 24–25, 183, 184
Mood control, 121–40
Moore, J., 187
Morris, P. E., 194
Morris, R. J., 198
Motivation, 122–23
Mullen, B., 187
Muñoz, R. F., 192

Nadel, L., 197
Nathan, R. S., 192
Necker Cube, 111–14
Negation. *See* Denial
Negative thoughts, 128–38
Nemeroff, C., 182
Network model, 51, 124
Neuberg, S. L., 191
Newcomb, T. M., 189
Nisbett, R. E., 185
Norcross, J. C., 182

Object language, 48–49
Oblivion, 73–76
Obsession, 5–7, 20–21
  abnormal and normal, 6
  and depression, 127
  synthetic, 161–80
  traumatic, 162–67, 174
Opportunity structures, 90
Optimism, 139
Orderliness, 21, 85–88

Pace, L. F., 186
Page, M., 195
Pain, 62–65

Paradoxical intention, 175–76
Parallel processes, 55–56
Parks, G. A., 183
Payne, D., 182
Pelham, B. W., 187
Pennebaker, James W., 36, 182,
  184, 194, 196, 198
Pershod, D., 182
Person perception, 80–82
Phobia, 5, 7, 154–55, 176–77,
  194
Pichot, P., 192
Plutchik, R., 191
Polivy, J., 182, 183
Pope, K. S., 185
Positive feedback system, 169–70,
  197–98
Positive mood, 138
Positive self-distracters, 134
Posner, M. I., 182
Posttraumatic stress disorder, 7
Posture, 14
Powers, W. T., 197
Predmore, S. C., 189
Prejudice, 117–20
Preoccupation, 4, 9–10, 168–69.
  See also Obsession
Problem solving, 127
Procrastination, 58
Program, computer, 41–43
Prohaska, M. L., 188
Pruzinsky, T., 186

Questions, 100–3
Quine, W. V., 184

Rachman, S. J., 181, 183, 184,
  185, 197